Praise for Molly Roden Winter's

More

"Very frank—and very hot. . . . *More* is bound to be passed furtively from friend to friend and gobbled up after the kids go to bed. It will make for an electrifying book club pick, inciting debate over what marriage means. . . . This book will no doubt find its way into the hands of many people who wouldn't be caught dead with a copy of *The Ethical Slut* but who are curious enough about open marriage to read the guidebook first, even if they're not quite ready to take the trip."   —*The Washington Post*

"Jaw-droppingly blunt. . . . I listened to the whole thing in a single sitting."   —Vulture

"[*More*] recounts the story of Ms. Winter's open marriage, detailing how she and her husband navigate the challenges, jealousies and joys of non-monogamy while exploring who they are as a couple and as individuals."   —*The New York Times*

"This memoir reads like a novel narrated in the first person—impossible to put down. . . . What will really captivate readers, however, is Winter's journey of introspection, a quest to understand herself and her needs and to find self-love and self-acceptance. Through her easily accessible, quickly devoured narrative, readers become something like confidants to Winter, rather than voyeurs. An honest look at how an open marriage can work, an excellent read for people interested in self-discovery or ethical non-monogamy."   —*Library Journal* (starred review)

MOLLY RODEN WINTER

More

Molly Roden Winter was raised in Evanston, Illinois, and lives in
Park Slope, Brooklyn, with her husband and two sons. Her personal essays have appeared in *The Cut, Time, Romper,* and elsewhere. She is half of the guitar-playing, songwriting duo House of
Mirth. Her website is mollyrodenwinter.com.

MORE

A MEMOIR
OF OPEN MARRIAGE

MOLLY RODEN WINTER

Vintage Books
A Division of Penguin Random House LLC
New York

FIRST VINTAGE BOOKS EDITION 2025

Published in the United States by Vintage Books, a division of Penguin Random House LLC, New York, and distributed in Canada by Penguin Random House Canada Limited, Toronto. Originally published in hardcover in the United States by Doubleday, a division of Penguin Random House LLC, New York, in 2024.

Vintage and colophon are registered
trademarks of Penguin Random House LLC.

The Library of Congress has cataloged the Doubleday edition as follows:
Names: Roden Winter, Molly, author.
Title: More: a memoir of open marriage / by Molly Roden Winter.
Description: First edition. | New York: Doubleday, 2024
Identifiers: LCCN 2022053109
Subjects: LCSH: Roden Winter, Molly. | Open marriage. | Non-monogamous
    relationships. | Sexual ethics. | Self-actualization (Psychology)
Classification: LCC HQ980 .R64 2024 | DDC 306.84/23—dc23
LC record available at https://lccn.loc.gov/2022053109

Vintage Books Trade Paperback ISBN: 978-0-593-46963-7
eBook ISBN: 978-0-385-54946-2

Book design by Maria Carella

vintagebooks.com

Printed in the United States of America
1st Printing

For Stewart

———

The erotic is the nurturer . . . of all our deepest knowledge.

—Audre Lorde

Author's Note

When I first conceived of writing this book, I consulted my old journals and was shocked to discover how often I had lied to myself. I understood, then, that I would have to do a great deal of emotional work to find a deeper truth than any I had previously written down. This book is my attempt to retrieve such truth.

That said, memory is imperfect. And stories are always written by preferencing one detail over another. In addition, I've changed most but not all names and modified many identifying details in order to protect the privacy of those involved. Sequence has sometimes shifted in deference to narrative cohesion.

Overall, though, I have rendered (my version of) the truth to the best of my ability.

MORE

PROLOGUE

MOM? ARE YOU THERE?

Mom? Where are you?

Mom, I need to talk to you.

Mom, please call me.

When the plane from LaGuardia touches down in Houston, I take my phone out of airplane mode and watch texts pile up like a deck of cards.

Text from Daniel, text from Daniel, from Daniel, from Daniel, from Daniel . . .

Mom, are you and Dad in an open marriage?

This is not Plan A. This is not even Plan W. This is, to put it mildly, cause for panic.

I follow the course of action I always take when faced with an unsolvable dilemma. I reach out to my husband, Stewart.

First, I take a screenshot of the texts. Underneath, I write, *WTF?! What should I do?*

Shit, he writes back. *Do you want to call me?*

I stumble off the plane, looking frantically for a place to collect myself—my water bottle and plane garbage, my thoughts and dignity. I find a spot against the wall, flanked by departure and arrival information boards.

The phone doesn't ring before Stew picks up.

"Oh, baby," he says. The sympathy in his voice reaches me through the phone. Stew knows how much I don't want to have this conversation with Daniel. He makes me an offer that's hard to refuse: "How about if *I* call him?"

"No, I'm the one he's asking. Maybe some TV show put the idea in his head and I can wriggle out of it."

"He's a mature kid. It'll be fine no matter what. I can talk to him later, too, okay?"

"Okay, thanks."

"I love you, my baby." And after sixteen years of marriage—after everything we've been through—I know in my marrow that this is true.

"I love you, too. Wish me luck."

"You don't need luck. You'll do great."

I lean back against the cool plaster wall, my carry-on suitcase squeezed between my legs, and prepare to call my child to discuss my sex life. People in various stages of flight continue to rush past. It's hard to hear—as much from the whoosh of blood in my ears as from the general airport hubbub.

I put the phone to one ear and my finger in the other.

"Hi, Daniel. Sorry, I just got your texts. I was on a flight. I'm in Houston."

My tone is casual, but I'm shaking.

"Hi," he replies. His voice, once so familiar but now with hardly an echo of his boyish squeak, startles me. "So—are you and Dad in an open marriage?"

Just like that.

Advice I received several years ago, when I drew the short straw and had to teach sixth-grade Health, rises to the surface of my brain: *Find out what they already know.*

"Wow. That's a big question. Why do you ask?"

Before I can congratulate myself on this brilliant gambit, Daniel responds.

"I saw Dad's OkCupid profile on his laptop, and that's what it said."

"Oh." I pause to scratch my calf with my instep, as if I could erase the discomfort rushing through me. And then, foolishly, I violate the other tenet of Health-teacher wisdom and offer up information without being asked.

"I want you to know something, Daniel," I say. "Dad and I are very happy together, and we're always honest with each other. He tells me everything, and I tell him everything."

On the other end of the line, Daniel is quiet for a beat. I want to believe he's ruminating on his good fortune at having such progressive, ethical parents. And then:

"Wait. You do it, too?"

I hold my breath. Daniel has seen Stewart's dating profile, but he hasn't seen mine. I realize too late that I misread the anxiety in his texts, in his newly minted man-voice. He thought his father was cheating on me. This call was meant to warn me, to protect his innocent mother from a betrayal measured in adolescent abstractions. But thinking your dad is committing adultery is worse than knowing your mother sleeps with other men, right? In this moment, I can't be sure. My brain floods with the myriad ways in which awareness of his mother's sexuality might damage a boy forever.

And then I exhale.

There comes a time when what you feared simply happens. I have dreaded this moment for seven years. Or maybe longer. Maybe I've dreaded it ever since Daniel was born and I realized that my child would one day grow up and see me with a critical eye, would know who I really am. But such a thing never happens in just a day; falling from grace can take a while. It took many years for me to see my own mother as a flawed, flesh-and-blood woman, a sexual and spiritual being with needs of her own that sometimes ran counter to those of her child.

And in the split second it takes to decide what to say next to Daniel, whether to tell the truth or a lie, I think of my mother. I wonder if she'd do it all differently now.

I wonder if I'd do it differently, too.

PART ONE

CHAPTER 1

THE RAIN POUNDS DOWN as Matt unlocks his door, pushes it open, and tumbles in behind me. I'm holding his jacket over my head, and as I lower it, a sheet of water slides onto the tiled floor. We're already in the kitchen. There's no foyer in his small studio apartment, no mudroom with four identical cubbies like I have in my house.

Matt is the one who's dripping wet, but he grabs a dish towel and offers it to me.

"I'm fine," I say. I can see little beads of water clinging to his curly hair, a single droplet at the tip of his nose. Instead of wiping them away, he tosses the towel onto the counter.

We face each other, in the small space between the oven and the sink. Over his shoulder, I can see his bed. At any moment, he could pick me up and carry me to it.

The hum of the refrigerator stops, and the sound of the rain is magnified. Matt is looking at me now with a concentrated intensity. His eyes are as steady as the center of a flame.

One of us—maybe both of us—says, "We shouldn't do this."

I know why Matt shouldn't. He's cheating on his girlfriend. But why shouldn't I?

What will this mean for you, Molly?

I lunge toward him, my hands buried in his thick hair, his long fingers grabbing my waist and pulling me in. And then his mouth covers mine. I feel the kiss of another man, someone other than Stewart. He tastes like beer and his lips are warm, softer than I expected, more pliable, so different from Stewart's kisses, which come in two flavors. There are the hello and good-bye kisses, which last only an instant and land on my lips like a rubber stamp of approval. And there are the kisses that come before sex, and during. Kisses that let me know that Stew is in control, that all I have to do is give myself over to him, follow him into whatever comes next, and all will be well.

In Matt's kiss, I feel something new. An invitation to take charge. To not wait for him to carry me but, instead, to take his hand and lead the way. I've anticipated this moment for so long, and now that it's here, my fear and longing do battle. It is the force of this longing—the high tide of my desire—that I fear the most. I open my eyes just as Matt opens his, and we each take a step back.

"I should go," I say. I leave him there, his eyes on me but the rest of him not moving to stop me. *This is all up to you,* his eyes say.

Out on the sidewalk, the storm is raging and I cannot think. My body is electric, and the water sends a current through me, leaves my mind insensate. I am nothing more than breath and blood and assembled pinpricks of sensation. I put one foot in front of the other—slowly, slowly. If I can delay my walk home, I can delay the end of this feeling. I can delay reentry into my life as the Wiper of Noses, the Doer of Dishes, the Nag in Residence.

I duck under an awning, reach for my phone, and stare blankly at it. I cannot make this decision alone. My thumbs type a torrent of words, and I hit Send. I've written a message to Stewart, and I need his reply to be faster than my feet. I've told him what I've done, what I want to do, and I've asked his permission.

Should I go back?

———

IT'S BEEN ALMOST TWO years since I first saw Matt, but I can hardly remember the before times, when I wasn't caught in a constant swirl of secret lust and mother's guilt.

The day I meet him is like any other. That morning, Stewart tells me he'll be home "early"—that is, early enough to find me awake but not early enough to help put the kids to bed.

Now it's 8:47 p.m. On what planet is this considered early?

I hear Stew's key in the door, and my body tenses. I won't give him a hello. My mouth won't do it.

"I need to get out," I say. I barely look at him for fear I'll scream, strike him, or worse.

"Where are you going?" he asks, perplexed. To him, "early" nights mean ordering dinner, watching TV together, hopefully sex.

"For a walk." I grab my jacket and keys. "I want to check on the house."

I'm through the door before he closes it.

Outside, a fine mist hovers in the lilac-scented air. I gulp at it as I walk, eyes on my feet, trying to slow my breath and release the constriction in my throat.

"Molly?"

I look up and recognize a teaching colleague from what feels like another lifetime.

"Kayla!" I say. "Sorry, I didn't see you there. I was in my own world, I guess."

"No worries." She reaches out to hug me. "It's been forever! What are you up to tonight?"

"Just walking. I had to get out. The kids drove me crazy today." Kayla is single. Childless. Beyond scenes of harried stay-at-home moms from sitcoms, I wonder if she has any idea what I'm talking about. But she looks at me sympathetically.

"You should come out with me! I'm going to meet some friends at the Gate."

I take in Kayla's smile, her high-heeled boots, her fresh lipstick and light perfume. I become conscious of my own appearance. I brushed my hair and slapped on deodorant this morning—some fifteen hours ago—but I certainly didn't shower. I'm wearing a hoodie, jeans, sneakers, and no makeup. I feel unbearably tired.

I look down at myself and realize something else. "I forgot my wallet," I tell her.

"Don't worry about it. I'll buy you a drink," she says, hooking her arm through mine. "Come on. You look like you need one."

I've walked past the Gate many times, pushing Daniel and then Nate in a stroller on my way to the playground across the street, but as we enter through the big wooden doors, I realize I've never set foot inside. Daniel was born just a week after we moved to Brooklyn, and I certainly haven't gotten a chance to explore the bar scene in the six years that have passed since.

As my eyes adjust to the dim light, I absorb the sounds of conversation, laughter, and Pearl Jam. I inhale the smells of beer and old wood and let my weight sink into the sticky floor. I've forgotten how relaxing it is to be in a place where children aren't allowed to enter.

Next to me, Kayla scans the room. When she spots her friends at a table in the back, she grabs my elbow and steers me toward them.

"Hi, guys! This is my friend Molly. I found her wandering the streets."

Two women at the end of the table smile and wave. I pull out the chair next to Kayla and sit, hanging my hoodie on the back.

"Molly, huh?" I hear a deep voice say. "I used to have a dog named Molly."

"I get that a lot." I look up to find the owner of the voice. Green, laughing eyes are staring into mine.

"I'm Matt," the voice continues. "What are you drinking?"

"Do they have an IPA?" I pause. "But I don't have any money. Kayla was going to loan me some."

"Don't worry about it." Matt waves a dismissive hand, standing up. He is lanky and tall, well over six feet. "One IPA coming up. I'll be right back." He heads to the bar.

To my left, Kayla is engaged in conversation with the rest of the group. I pretend to listen as my eyes dart to the right, to Matt. His back is to me, and I note the slim hips, the easy way he wears his jeans, his thick, curly hair, which stands up a little on top. My body reacts to what I see before my mind has time to catch up. A pleasant flutter has developed deep within my stomach, spreading up to my pounding heart and rushing down to my groin.

Matt turns around, holding two beers, and catches me staring. He grins as I look down at my hands on the table. My fingernails are short and stubby—I haven't had a manicure in months—and my wedding band glints in the bar light. I slip my hands onto my lap and, without touching the glass, slurp from the beer Matt has placed in front of me.

"Mmm," I say. "I haven't had a beer on tap in a while. Thanks."

"No problem," he says, an amused look still in his eyes. "I'm just curious. How did you end up getting dragged here? Where did Kayla find you?"

"I escaped from the asylum."

Matt laughs. "No offense, but that's pretty close to what I was going to guess. You have the air of an escapee." He takes a sip of beer and looks at me expectantly.

"I have two kids," I say, regretting my words immediately. It was nice not to be seen as a mother for all of five minutes. And this guy is too young to be a parent. "They're great, but they make me nuts sometimes. I had to get out, so I bolted without thinking about where I was going."

He nods. "I get that. I mean, not from personal experience, but my sister has two kids. She lives back in Iowa, but I spent a lot of time with her and my nieces last Christmas. That's probably how I recognized the look on your face."

"It's that obvious, huh?" I feel my shoulders relax. I feared my confession of having a family would open a gulf between us. But Matt's words have reassured me.

"Not in a bad way at all," he says. "You just look like someone who needs to decompress."

I hold up my glass. "Cheers to that."

"Cheers," says Matt as we clink our glasses.

The hours and beers pass like a montage from an '80s movie. In one clip, Matt celebrates with me as my dart hits the target. In another, I stand out front with the cool kids, taking a drag on a cigarette and petting someone's dog. Finally, there I am back at the table, saying to Matt as the group gathers their things to go, "I owe you a few rounds." And then, like a director trying to help an ingénue get into character, I urge myself on. "You live around here, right? Give me your number and we'll do this again sometime." *Bravo!*

"I'll give you mine if you give me yours," he answers. "I'm gonna hold you to your offer."

"Hey, Kayla, do you have a pen?" I ask. "Teachers always have pens," I explain to Matt.

Kayla reaches into her purse and pulls out a pen, surveying me with raised eyebrows.

"See? It's even red."

I scrawl my number on a napkin, then hand the pen to Matt and he does the same. Kayla looks from him to me and then whispers in my ear, "I guess I didn't have to pay for your drinks after all."

I look at her sideways and whisper back, "I'm married, Kayla. It's nothing."

"If you say so." She doesn't sound convinced.

As I walk home, touching the bar napkin in my pocket, the cool air has a sobering effect. I stop to consider what I've done. I exchanged numbers with a man. A younger man. An unmarried man. I review what I know about him. He's from Iowa—a state I've crossed in the back seat of a station wagon more times than I can count, on the way to visit my mom's parents in Denver. He went to college with Kayla, so he must be about her age, which is eight years younger than I am. He has a sister and nieces with whom he is close. He works in Manhattan, doing what I'm still not sure. He is funny, sweet, a good listener—and gorgeous. He knows I'm married, and he still wants to go out for drinks with me again. At least he says he does. The balloon in my chest deflates a bit. I probably won't hear from him again. But even so, I had a great time. One of the best nights I've had since my children were born, in fact.

My children.

I have a sudden urge to see them, to hug Daniel, to hold Nate. In part, this is driven by a pang of guilt for the hours I've spent without them on my mind. But it's more, too. I love being a mother. I know this is true. Even on the worst days, when they were both still in diapers and neither of them napped, when Stewart was at work and the idea of a shower was a distant dream, I'd call my mother from a prostrate position on the living room floor. I'd watch the chaos of flying Cheerios and listen to epic dramas unfold between Diesel the Villain and Thomas the Hero, and my mom would ask me: *But even if you could, would you trade places with Stewart?* And I'd have to acknowledge that I wouldn't. For then I would miss the sticky kisses and the victorious poops in potties, the joy of watching Daniel patiently teach Nate the arbitrary rules of his Thomas the Tank Engine games. I would miss the bubble baths and the belly laughs and the thousands of ways that motherhood nearly breaks my heart with love every day, even as I fantasize about running as fast as I can away from it all.

I quicken my pace toward home, pulling my keys from my pocket as I walk. When I step through the front door, I notice the toys, shoes, and jackets strewn across the living room floor, exactly where they'd been discarded earlier in the evening. I sigh, sidestepping the mess. It will still be there tomorrow.

I creep into the boys' room first. I listen to their breathing and inhale their scent. I kiss each of them on the forehead and study their faces, expressive even in sleep. Daniel's brow is furrowed, serious as always. Nate, meanwhile, has a smile at the edges of his lips, as though he's cooking up a dream full of mischief.

I'm not surprised to see the light on in our bedroom. Stewart often stays awake until two or three in the morning, and though I feel like I've been gone for ages, it's just after midnight. I open the door to find Stew sitting up in bed, reading one of the music industry magazines that I constantly find on the floor and pile on his piano stool.

"Look who's back," he says. "I thought you'd be home in less than an hour. I would have called but you left your phone." He holds it up as proof.

"Sorry," I say, rushing past him into the bathroom. "I have to pee." I pull down my jeans and sit on the toilet with the door open. It will be easier to talk if I don't have to look at him.

"So where were you? I was getting worried."

"I didn't even make it to 10th Street. I ran into Kayla, and we went out for a few drinks."

"Kayla?"

"One of my teaching friends." Stewart had rarely accompanied me to school functions, but I feel a need to keep talking, so I add, "I can't believe you never met her."

"Then who's Matt?"

"Matt?" I ask, trying to sound casual and buying time with a strategic flush of the toilet. "He went to college with Kayla. He was out at the bar with us. How do you know about him?" I walk out of the bathroom with my fingers held tightly together. If I start to chew on my cuticles, Stew will spot my tell.

"He sent you a text a few minutes ago," says Stewart, gesturing to my phone.

"What did it say?"

He flips it open and clears his throat, lowering his voice to a sexy baritone: *"Great meeting you tonight, Molly. I hope we can do it again soon. —Matt."* He looks at me, waiting.

"Like I said, he was at the bar with us." I busy myself with untying my shoelaces to avoid Stewart's gaze. "I forgot my wallet, so I flirted my way into a couple free drinks."

"It looks like you did an excellent job," he says. I can feel his eyes on my face, which has started to color. "So are you going to see him again?"

"Of course not," I say, pulling off my socks.

"Why not?"

I glance over at him. It's been a while, but I've seen that look before. "Because I'm married. To you. Remember?"

"I remember."

"And we have kids now. And Matt is young and single and definitely not interested."

"He sounds interested to me." He watches me as I unhook my bra. "Seeing his text made me pretty crazy, actually."

I pause to consider this. Before we had kids, Stewart and I had sex at least three times a week—occasionally three times a day. Lately, we've been lucky to have sex twice a month. Or rather, *he's* been lucky. As if conforming to every cliché I've heard about married sex, I'm too tired to be interested. I treat sex like one more wifely obligation. And Stew feels it. In response, he tries to mix it up, to do new things, to kiss me or lick me in a new way, to hold me down or slide a finger into my asshole. But all I want is a quickie, a tried-and-true method for a fast-tracked mutual orgasm that will get me to sleep a few precious hours before I hear Nate's cries.

"Baby, I'm glad you're enjoying this. But it's not gonna happen."

"I disagree," he says as I climb into bed. "It'll happen if you want it to happen. So I've decided."

"Decided what?"

"You can go out with him again. As long as you tell me every-thing." He pulls me toward him, making me the little spoon, and kisses me on the back of my head.

That night, as I lie next to Stewart, I can't sleep. My mind jumps from Matt to Stew and back again.

I hope we can do it again soon.

You can go . . . as long as you tell me everything.

I think about a conversation Stewart and I had before we were even engaged. The topic was our respective number of sexual part-ners, and the huge gulf between my number and his. I'd had four; he'd had dozens. Then Stew made a prediction. How unlikely and dangerous it had seemed to me at the time.

"Just wait," he'd said. He looked so much like my celebrity crush—the tennis player Andre Agassi, with that round bald head and brown eyes, doelike but naughty. "Ten years from now, you're gonna see some guy and you'll wonder what it'd be like to fuck him. And it's okay with me. You just have to tell me about it."

And here we are. Ten years later.

CHAPTER 2

THE NEXT TWO WEEKS feel like four. This is because I've split neatly in half in order to live a double life.

In one life, I wake with the kids at dawn, make breakfast and pack lunches, manage pickups and playdates, cook dinner and run baths, read bedtime stories and sing lullabies. I greet Stewart when he comes home late in the evening, give backrubs or make love, and sleep by his side. I am the picture of the dutiful mother and wife—but only in service to my other life, the one where I think about Matt. I picture what he's doing and who he's with. I wonder if he's thinking about me, too. Even after sex with Stew, I touch myself and imagine it is Matt, bringing me to orgasm again.

After the text he sent on the night we met, I forced myself to wait until the following afternoon to write him back. Since then, we've exchanged a handful of messages, each one I receive sending me into a frenzy until I've answered with as much casualness as I can muster. Then I wait in agony for the next text to arrive.

How was your weekend? from Matt on Sunday night, answered by my *Not bad—yours?* on Monday morning.

Pretty chill. Gotta busy week tho arrives on Monday night, signaling me to wait a few days, until I can't stand it anymore and respond with *Hope you're surviving!*

We go on like this until the middle of the next week. When

Matt answers one of my inanities with *I could use a beer,* I take it as my opening.

Well you know, I do owe you a couple of those, I write. I gnaw at my nails as I await his reply. This time, it comes within an hour.

Yeah, you do. When are you free?

In bed with Stew that night, I skip over my own part in the text thread and say, "Matt asked me to get a drink with him."

"Yeah?" Stew says, as if he's expected this all along. His hand instinctively reaches for my thigh under the covers. "And what did you say?"

"I didn't answer yet."

"Baby, I'm into it. I promise."

"Are you sure?" I turn on my side to face him while keeping his hand sandwiched between my legs.

He kisses my neck, moves his other hand to my breast. "I'm sure."

I envy his certainty.

The next day, with Daniel at school and Nate smearing bananas on the kitchen table, I text Matt. It's taken me hours of mental composition to come up with the perfect message. *What are you doing on Friday?* feels too inquisitive. *Are you available on Friday?* is too formal. *Let's go out on Friday!* is too desperate.

The worst part is, I can't ask anyone for advice. Most of my friends are married. I picture myself saying, *But Stewart* wants *me to go out with him,* and the look of disbelief on their faces.

How about Friday?

I look at the three words on the screen. Casual but confident, I think, and hit Send. I don't have to wait for Matt's reply.

You're on.

THE DAYS LEADING TO Friday pass in a blur. I tell Stew I'm arranging for a babysitter so he can stay late at work. The real reason is that the thought of him getting home even one minute late makes my chest tighten. More than that, I want to be alone when I get home from seeing Matt. I will need to be alone.

On Friday, I discover I can't eat. On a typical day, I gobble up the rest of Nate's scrambled eggs for breakfast and eat crusts of grilled cheese or hot dog remnants for lunch, snacks of Veggie Booty and granola bars all afternoon. But today, even coffee feels like a bad idea, so I sip at a Starbucks venti iced tea. When that's gone, I chew a hole in the straw.

The babysitter arrives at five thirty, giving me over an hour to shower and get dressed. I grab a Corona and a bottle opener and hide them under my sweatshirt as I scurry to the bedroom. As I take a long swig, my phone buzzes. A text from Stew.

Have fun tonight, baby. I'll be thinking about you.

Something about his message irritates me. Does he think this is all for him?

At a quarter to seven, I'm ready to leave. Daniel is absorbed in *SpongeBob,* but Nate screams and cries as he watches me head for the door.

"He's fine," the babysitter assures me after I hug and kiss Nate for the third time. "Let's go pick some toys for the bath," I hear her say as I close the door behind myself.

He's fine, I repeat inwardly, standing on the sidewalk in front of our apartment. *He's fine, he's fine, he's fine.*

I remember encountering a line from Kate Chopin's *The Awakening,* back when I rode the subway alone on my way to work and had time to read. Edna, the heroine, says this: "I would give my life for my children; but I wouldn't give myself." I was confused by the distinction. But now that I have kids, it makes more sense. Still, one quandary remains: Who is my "self" if not a mother and a wife?

I honestly don't know. Perhaps it's time to find out.

———

MATT AND I ARE meeting at the Gate again, and my hands tremble as I pull open the heavy door and search the room. I see him sitting at the bar in jeans and a button-down. When he smiles and waves, the tension drains from my body and is replaced by something else. Something strong and unmistakable.

Desire.

I walk toward him as he stands up. I'd forgotten how tall he is. Stewart always accuses me of having a type—tall and slim, with a full head of hair. *Just picture the opposite of me and that's what you're into,* he's said more than once.

Without thinking, I do what feels natural. I put my arms around Matt, my face level with a triangle of exposed skin, and squeeze. This could be a friendly hug, I think, not actually caring. I inhale his smell—soap and beer and youth and freedom—and realize he's squeezing me too. We hold on for an extra beat.

"Hey there," says Matt, looking down at me with his sea-green eyes.

"Hey," I say.

I take off my jacket as he keeps his eyes on me. "You clean up pretty good."

I laugh. "Yeah, I actually took a shower and put on clothes without stains."

I say this casually, but in truth, I spent hours thinking about what to wear. I didn't want to look like I was trying too hard, but I also wanted to replace the image in his mind's eye of a disheveled mom. I'm wearing black jeans, boots, and a form-fitting sweater. I've got on makeup and hoop earrings and have blow-dried my hair. Sitting on a barstool next to Matt, I feel pretty. Pretty like Stewart made me feel when we first started dating. I know it's not Stew's fault that my self-image is in the toilet. He tells me all the time that I'm beautiful. But it's hard to believe him. Motherhood drained the pretty out of me. I forgot how good it feels.

"You want the IPA again?" he asks. "This pilsner is good, too, if you want to try it." He slides his beer along the bar toward me.

I pick it up and take a sip. My lips are on the same glass his lips touched. He remembers the beer I drank last time.

"Delicious. But I'm supposed to be buying *your* drinks tonight."

"Don't worry. I'll let you get the next round or two."

As we drink our beers, it's hard to concentrate. I only half listen as we engage in small talk, expanding on the personal data we exchanged at our first meeting. Mostly, I'm aware of how close our faces are to each other. The fact that our knees keep touching. Did he consider this when he chose seats at the bar? That we wouldn't have a table creating a boundary between our bodies?

It isn't until I've almost finished my second beer that I become acutely aware of Matt's words. I've asked how long he's lived in Park Slope, a seemingly innocuous question.

"My girlfriend and I just moved here a few months ago," he says. "We have a place on 16th Street. What about you and your husband?"

Girlfriend. Husband.

I pause. Of course he knows I'm married. I never tried to hide it. But hearing him say the word *husband* has brought Stew into the bar with us. And he has a girlfriend. Why does this information matter so much to me? Maybe he assumes we're both cheating. Maybe this is only friendship after all. I drain the rest of my beer and look toward the ceiling, as if calculating my answer to his question.

"Let's see," I say. "We moved right before Daniel was born, and he's six now, so yeah. Six years. We're moving to a house soon. Still in the Slope, so we plan to be here for good. We're going through renovations now. It's a huge ordeal but it'll be nice to have more space."

I listen to myself ramble and feel sick. I sound so pleased with my cookie-cutter life. *Daniel's six now. Moving to a house. Going through renovations. What an ordeal!* I want to gag. This isn't me. But neither is the person who's been touching knees and making googly eyes at a near stranger.

I pick up my phone, fingers fumbling.

"God, it's later than I thought," I say. "I should probably get home for the sitter."

"Oh, okay," says Matt. "Can I walk you?"

"No, it's in the other direction. But once we move to 10th Street, we'll be neighbors!" I chirp, trying to sound extra neighborly. I pull some bills from my wallet and put them under the empty pint glass. "Here's for the beer. This was fun!" I nearly jump off the barstool and am now jamming my arms into my jacket.

"Yeah it was," says Matt, looking puzzled. "Get home safe."

"I will!" I wave as I wriggle between the twentysomethings who stand between me and the door, blocking my escape. "Bye!"

Outside, I turn the corner and head for the shadows of Third Street. What am I doing? What was I thinking? I am a wife. A mother with young children. How did I think a "date" with a younger guy would go? I pick up my pace toward home. Of course he has a girlfriend. Is he supposed to pine for me during the weeks I'm with my family, saving himself for beers at the bar with me? He probably just finds me entertaining, an older woman who slobbers over him and boosts his ego.

I pull out my phone and send a text to Stewart: *On my way home now.*

Already? he writes back. I can picture him, holding his phone, waiting for a salacious update so he can jerk off in his office. I see his face falling when he realizes no sexy details are on the way.

Yeah. It didn't feel right.

Oh, baby, I'm sorry. Are you okay? Should I come home?

I'm not okay. And the fact that Stewart knows it makes my tears rise to the surface. But how to explain? How can I tell him I need to lie in bed alone, to cry, to mourn the loss of something I never had in the first place?

I'm fine! I write, realizing too late that the exclamation point gives away my lie. *Just tired. Gonna go to sleep.*

Okay, he writes back. *I'm here if you want to talk. I love you.*

Thanks, baby. I love you, too.

But it's not enough, I think. Nothing will ever be enough again.

CHAPTER 3

I'M THINKING ABOUT MATT less and less. For the first few months after my failed "date," when Stew and I have sex, he tries to keep the fantasy of Matt alive. Talking about Matt feeds Stewart's libido. When he tells me to imagine what Matt's cock looks like, how his mouth would feel on my pussy, Stew gets rougher than I want him to be. Once, he calls me *cunt* during sex, and I start to cry.

"Are you mad at me?" I blubber.

"Oh, baby, no," Stewart says, holding me as I sniffle into his chest. "I don't mean it in a bad way. I like imagining you with other men. It's part of what turns me on. It's just that, if I don't figure out how to release some tension, I'll end up coming too soon."

But what works for Stewart doesn't work for me. It's not Matt's cock I want. Not really. It's his attention. I want to imagine Matt making dinner for me. How Matt might gaze at me the first time I stand naked before him. But those things feel outside the purview of Stewart's fantasy and therefore out of bounds.

"Let's not talk about him in bed anymore, okay?" I say. But instead of telling Stewart the truth—that Matt has revealed a void in my life, a need for something that marriage and motherhood cannot fill, and the mere mention of his name fills me with an ache, a longing I cannot bear—I say, "I just want to concentrate on *you* when we have sex." And I do my best to put Matt out of my mind.

There are plenty of distractions. We move into our new house, and I decide to go back to teaching. I tell Stew a small piece of the truth of what the Matt experience taught me: that I need a life outside the kids. I take a full-time job back at my old school and share a classroom with Kayla. Both boys are school-age now, too. I can live the dream of grabbing coffee with my colleagues, of going to the bathroom without a toddler following me, of using my brain for hours at a time.

And yet, most days I wake up when the sky is still dark, and by eight a.m., when Daniel and Nate have been deposited in their classrooms and I am in mine, I'm bathed in sweat, about to start a full day of wrangling adolescents. By five p.m., when I pick the boys up from Afterschool, I often have a migraine. With my eyes at half-mast, we take the subway home, and I make dinner and pack lunches for the next day, wash the dishes and do a load of laundry, get the kids bathed and into pajamas, read a story and sing songs as I tuck them in, maybe grade some papers, and by the time Stewart comes home—"early" as he still likes to call it—my fury bubbles through my skin like the surface of the sun.

But the upside is this: by living in a constant state of chaos, I can spend most of my time pretending everything is fine. And, sometimes, it is.

JUST AFTER SPRING break, I get an Evite message in my inbox:

SHHHHH! IT'S A SURPRISE!!!
LET'S CELEBRATE KAYLA'S BIRTHDAY!

Where: Sing Sing Karaoke on Avenue A
When: Friday, April 24, 2009
Time: 8 p.m.–????
RSVP here
And remember . . . DON'T TELL KAYLA!!!

I click the link with my heart racing and scan the list of invitees. There he is, at the very bottom: *Matthew Wolfe*. It must be him. And of course he has a sexy last name. Would my legs still be shaking if I'd seen *Matthew Dinkledorf* on the list? Maybe. He hasn't RSVP'd yet, but I tell myself it doesn't matter either way. Kayla is my friend. There's no question about whether I'm going to her party. I click *Attending* next to my name and ignore the *+1*. Stew won't want to go anyway. *Can't wait!* I write in the comments box.

Every day for the next two weeks, sometimes every hour, I click on the Evite link and check Matt's RSVP status. I'm not sure what would be worse, a *+1* next to his name or *Sorry, can't make it*. Meanwhile, I tell Stewart about the party, and when I say he doesn't have to go, he breathes a sigh of relief. He doesn't mention it again. Apparently, he's forgotten that Kayla is my connection to Matt, which makes me breathe my own sigh of relief. I don't think I could tolerate his innuendo.

Two days before the party, I check my email during a free period and find another message from Evite. *Don't forget to RSVP!* reads the subject line. Maybe this will spur Matt to action. I force myself to wait until after school to check. I usher the last students out of the classroom and angle my computer away from Kayla's desk. Two clicks, and there it is: *Matthew Wolfe: Attending*.

No *+1*.

I PLAN TO GO to Sing Sing with another teaching friend, but at the last minute, she cites a sore throat and bails. I'll have to arrive at the party alone. On the F train, I bounce a knee up and down like one of my seventh graders. As I walk along Houston Street, a lyric from a Liz Phair song runs through my head, over and over, in a dizzying loop.

Why can't I breathe whenever I think about you?

Everyone is supposed to be punctual so as not to ruin the surprise. I'm cutting it close, so taking a lap around the block to calm myself isn't an option. As I approach Sing Sing, I dart my eyes around, searching for Matt on the sidewalk.

Inside the front door, his height makes him easy to spot. He's at the front of the pack making its way into one of the larger private rooms. I catch his profile, laughing with his college friends, completely at ease. I've made a mistake. I shouldn't have come, especially not alone.

I duck into the bathroom, take a few deep breaths, and give myself a pep talk: *This isn't a big deal. It's a freaking party. You never get to go out. Just relax and have a good time.* I steady myself with a final look in the mirror and walk into the hallway. I can hear singing and laughter coming from each of the closed doors. As I enter Kayla's party room, the lyrics become distinct: *The only one who could ever reach me was the son of a preacher man.*

The room is dark, and the two women who'd been at the Gate last year are up front, under the rotating lights of a disco ball, screaming into microphones and dancing. Another cluster of people sit on the couch, studying the tomes of song choices by the light of a cell phone. I notice a table off to the side with pitchers of beer and start toward it. I need something to do with my hands. As I reach for a cup, I hear a deep voice behind me.

"Hey there. Could you pour me one too?"

I turn around and see Matt grinning at me, his eyes again laughing.

"Sure!" I say, grateful for a clear task. I pour a beer and hand it to him. When his fingers touch mine, a jolt of electricity rips through me. "How have you been?"

I concentrate on pouring another beer for myself, avoiding his gaze.

"I've been good, thanks. What about you?"

"Good, good," I babble, unsure of what else to say. I take a swallow of beer to stall, then look up. His eyes are so fucking green. I let myself sink into them for a moment, then look away.

"Are you planning to sing?" I gesture toward the microphones.

"Hell yeah," he says. "I have some standard karaoke numbers, and they kill every time. One of them's a duet, though, so I'm gonna need some help. Are you game?"

"I'd be honored," I say. How is it possible we're flirting again, that it's this easy? It's been over a year since I last saw him. And I'd acted like a moron. Now here we are, drinking beer and planning to take the stage together, like nothing ever happened. But nothing *did* happen, I remind myself.

Kayla makes her big entrance and is pulled up front for almost every song of the night. The hours fly past. It hardly matters who is holding a microphone, and the whole room constantly erupts into song. *Don't stop believin'! I like big butts and I cannot lie! Girls just wanna have fun!*

Matt makes sure I'm never with an empty cup for long, and when the lights abruptly flicker on, signaling the end of our prepaid hours, I watch the room spin around before it comes to rest at a slight tilt.

One of Kayla's friends, the woman who planned the party, stands on the couch, pushing her hair out of her eyes. "The party isn't over, guys! It would be great if you could each give me some cash for the room and then we'll go to the bar next door. 'Kay?"

Twenty-dollar bills fill the air as people grab their jackets, ready to party on into the night. I become aware of myself as something separate from the throng. Am I the oldest one here? Am I the only one with kids at home?

I hand over my twenty and turn to get my jacket. But Matt is already holding it.

"We still have to sing our duet," he says.

He is looking at me in a new way. Or am I imagining it? I think of Nate and Daniel, in their beds and asleep for the night.

As if he's reading my mind, he asks, "Or do you have to get home?"

I swallow. "Um, I can stay for a little while. But I think they cut off the room already."

"Yeah, but the small rooms are only ten bucks for a half hour after midnight." His face is close to mine, and his voice is almost a whisper. "Can you give me half an hour?"

He's planned this. Even done research. I manage to nod.

"Great. I'll be right back."

In a daze, I wander into the hallway and fumble with my phone. There's a text from Stewart, sent about an hour ago.

Hey, baby. I finished work a little early so I let the sitter go home. Stay out as long as you want and have fun! I love you.

I pause. Why didn't I tell Stew that Matt would be here? Why don't I want to tell him now? He likes the idea of my flirting with someone else—and more. So why do I feel like I'm crossing a line?

Thanks! Having a great time. Everyone's getting another drink at the bar but I won't be super late. I love you too.

I hit Send and look up. Matt is walking toward me.

"We're all set."

The rest of the group is already outside. I can hear a high-pitched drunken voice trying to convince the more sober party-goers to come to the bar. With no witnesses remaining, Matt grabs my hand and pulls me in the direction of door number three. The room is tiny. Inside, we fall onto the love seat in front of a screen. I feel the pressure of his long leg against mine, from hip to knee.

"Okay," he says. "Let me find it." He grabs a songbook from

the side table and scans the titles. "Here it is! You'd better get your mic." He punches the code into the remote control and stands with a dramatic cough.

I recognize the opening bars of "Islands in the Stream" and fake a groan as I stand up, too. "Your Iowa is showing, Matt."

"Don't pretend you don't love this song. Shut up and sing."

Matt croons the opening Kenny Rogers lines with his eyes closed. I await the pink lyrics to appear, cuing Dolly's entrance. As he sings, Matt steps behind me and wraps one arm around my waist, pulling me toward him.

> You do something to me that I can't explain
> Hold me closer and I feel no pain . . .

As we rock back and forth to the music, I try to concentrate. Not on the lyrics, but on the points of contact between his body and mine. He rests his chin on the top of my head, my butt fits neatly into his pelvis. I can feel his breath on my scalp, his diaphragm expanding and contracting against my back. A thread of sensation runs from my feet to my head, like the vibration of a one-stringed guitar. I think of a line from a book called *I Love Dick*, which I read when I first moved to the city. The book made me feel unsophisticated—I barely understood it—but also daring when people saw it in my hands on the subway.

"*Desire isn't lack, it's surplus energy—a claustrophobia inside your skin.*"

When the song ends, we put down our microphones, and Matt gives me a quick squeeze before removing his arm from its hold on my body. I turn around and look at him.

"Best ten bucks I ever spent," he says. If we are going to kiss, it will happen now. He is waiting for a signal from me. All I have to do is reach out and touch his arm, and he will do the rest. But I can't do it.

"I should get going," I say. And the moment is gone.

WHEN I ARRIVE HOME, I find Stewart watching TV on the couch.

"Home so soon? How was the party?"

"Fun!" I say, pulling off my jacket. "I'll tell you about it tomorrow. I'm beat." All I want to do is climb into bed and replay every moment of the night. I lean over the back of the couch to kiss him. It is a quick kiss, a perfunctory kiss.

"Okay," he says, studying me. "You look nice, by the way. I haven't seen you do your eyes like that in a while." There is a question in his tone, but I refuse to acknowledge it.

"Thanks. I'll see you in bed."

"I'll come with you." He turns off the TV. "I've seen this movie before."

Stewart lies on the bed, and I leave the bathroom door open. I keep my mouth busy with tooth brushing and forced yawns. But I feel a confession rising within me. It makes no sense to not tell him what happened.

Without really deciding, as Stew turns off the lights, I hear myself say, "Matt was there."

"I know."

I roll on my side to face him, my eyes wide in the dark. "You do? How?"

"Molly," he laughs, stroking my bare shoulder, "you're not hard to read. So what happened?"

As I replay the evening for Stew, I am only semi-aware of how I reframe events, shift to the edges of truth. In this version, Matt is the protagonist. I play the role of the object of his desire, not an active participant.

"He kept refilling my glass without my realizing how much I'd had to drink. . . . I promised to sing a duet with him, but I didn't think he'd hold me to it. . . . And before I knew what was happening, he put his arms around me. . . ."

As I speak, Stewart's hand moves over my body, stroking my hip, my ass. And when I finish my tale, he picks up the narrative.

"Do you know what Matt's doing right now?" He lets his fingers wander across my panties.

"No," I whisper.

"I do. He's thinking about what he wishes he'd done to you on that couch."

"What did he want to do?"

"This," Stewart says, pushing my underwear down and putting two fingers inside me.

I close my eyes. I am back on the love seat. I am opening my legs and letting Matt's long fingers roam, feeling my wetness.

"Fuck me," I say, for perhaps the first time in our married life. As Stewart enters me, I moan. And let myself be fucked by Matt.

THE NEXT AFTERNOON, a Saturday, I'm at my friend Jessie's house. A few years earlier, Jessie had a monster crush on her son's piano teacher. I was one of the few people she confided in. So as we drink coffee in the kitchen and our kids play in the next room, I decide to trust her.

"I have something to tell you," I say.

"A grown-up topic?" She puts an elbow on the table and rests her chin in her palm. "I'm all ears."

There's a thrill to sharing my secret, and I savor the look of captivation on Jessie's face as she listens. But when I get to the part about Matt putting his arms around me at karaoke, Jessie's expression changes. She starts to look *concerned*.

"Wait a sec," she says, holding up a hand to interrupt. "Are you planning to sleep with this guy?"

"Well, here's the thing," I continue, taking a deep breath. "Stewart *wants* me to sleep with him."

"What?" She shakes her head as if to wake herself from a crazy dream.

"He says the idea of it turns him on."

Jessie stares at me. She puts her interrupting hand, still hanging in the air, on my arm.

"Molly," she says. "I've got to be honest with you. It sounds like you're entering dangerous territory."

My throat starts to close. The part of my brain that has governed my life thus far agrees with her. What's happening with Matt feels *very* dangerous. This is why I'm telling Jessie about it, I realize. I'm hoping she will convince me that this feeling is worth the danger. That once in a while, it's important to do the dangerous thing. Otherwise, you might get suffocated by your own sense of safety. You might wake up one morning and find yourself tucked inside the Tupperware with the leftover chicken and carrot sticks you packed for everyone else's lunch, and there's no way out, no entry point for air.

I'm relieved to hear crying in the next room.

"Stop it, Nate! Mom! Nate is messing up our train tracks again!"

"To be continued," says Jessie as we stand up and move toward the cries.

As I leave Jessie's house later that afternoon, she hands me a piece of paper with a name and a phone number.

"I'm not telling you what to do," she says as I wrangle Nate into his jacket, "but I used to see this therapist in the city. He's awesome. You might want to talk about this whole Matt thing with someone."

Jessie gives me a quick hug, and I head out with my kids, keeping my expression as neutral as I can, my emotions vacuum-packed.

IT TAKES ME A while to make an appointment. This is my second attempt at therapy since arriving in New York. My first summer in the city, I lived with Nina, my childhood best friend, who'd gone to Barnard. The year prior, when I broke up with my college boyfriend, William, after following him upstate, I spent most weekends visiting Nina in Manhattan. She listened to all my William-inspired woes, supplied me with a ready-made group of friends, and even got me an interview at the school where she'd done a psychology internship. I got the job, moved in with Nina, and then had to figure out how to spend my endless hours of "vacation" before the school year began. Each day, at least one of these hours was occupied by crying.

"Let me find you a therapist," Nina said one day when she came home from work and saw me still in bed, used tissues piled in my lap as I watched *Casablanca* on the VCR. "Trust me. *Everyone* in New York is in therapy."

I brought a giant corn muffin with me to my first appointment, alternately crying about William and nibbling at it throughout the session. At the end, my new therapist looked disdainfully at the crumbs I'd dropped on my chair and asked me not to eat during future sessions. After that, I strove to make a better impression, keeping my hunger as well as my feelings in check. For the duration of the school year, I trekked to the Upper East Side once a week and made what I hoped were sage comments about how well I was handling my adjustment to a new job and city.

One day, my therapist came out of her office and into the

waiting area where I sat, looked me straight in the eye, and held out her hand.

"Hello. I'm Dr. Randolph," she said. I'd been talking to her every week for a year—close to fifty times—and she didn't know who I was.

But now, on a Wednesday at four o'clock, while my kids are in Afterschool, I find myself seated on a narrow couch, flanked by decorative pillows, in the office of Mitchell Kaplan, licensed therapist. Right away, I can tell that Mitchell is not another Dr. Randolph. His age is difficult to determine. He has a full head of white hair but a young face and electric-blue eyes. His name lets me know he's Jewish, while his accent reveals him to be a fellow Midwesterner—a combination that immediately makes me feel at home. The impeccable cut of his clothing, coupled with his tendency to gesture broadly, makes me suspect he's gay. He also asks me to call him by his first name. In other words, Mitchell is perfect.

I spend almost forty minutes telling him my story. He interrupts only to ask clarifying questions. When I finish, I look at him expectantly, knowing that I hope to get from Mitchell the same thing I wanted from Jessie.

I want to sleep with Matt. I don't want to be stopped. I want to be given permission.

Mitchell does neither. Instead, he asks, "What will this mean for you, Molly? Why do you want to sleep with him?"

I pause, trying to grasp the scope of his question. "I don't know," I admit.

"Well," says Mitchell, leaning forward in his chair like a co-conspirator, "people have been having sex for centuries without understanding why they do it. But here's my suggestion."

I lean forward, too, barely able to breathe.

"I think you and I should spend some time figuring it out."

As I leave Mitchell's office, having made another appointment

in two weeks' time, I feel like I've put down one burden and lifted
another. I have a glimmer of awareness, like an aura on the edge of
my peripheral vision, foretelling the onset of a migraine.

My obsession with Matt isn't about him. It's about me.

THE NEXT SATURDAY MORNING, I sit on the floor next to the
bathtub where Nate splashes and plays. I've discovered that giving
Nate an early morning bath allows me an extra half hour of rest,
if not sleep. With a second cup of coffee at my side, I lean my head
against the tiled wall and close my eyes.

My phone vibrates with a new text. It's from Matt. It's the first
time he's written me since the karaoke party, and my heart lurches
into my throat.

Hey there. What are you doing later?

I wait a moment, then write back: *Probably taking the kids to
the playground. Why?*

No, I mean later later. Like tonight, after they go to bed.

Mitchell's words come rushing back. *What will this mean for
you, Molly?* I'm supposed to figure it out first, right?

I chew my finger as I consider how to respond to Matt. I've
been chewing my finger a lot in recent days. The skin around my
nail bed is red and angry. Accusatory.

What did you have in mind? I write.

*Would you be up for a drink? There's a bar near my place I've been
wanting to try. Maybe 9:00?*

I can hear Stewart through the bathroom wall, recording in
his studio. He plays the same five notes over and over again, creating one of his short compositions of promo music that are "favors"
for clients, extra work that always seems to consume our weekends.
I could go ask him right now. Our only plan for the night is to

order takeout. I'm sure he'd love to send me on a date with Matt afterward. But I don't want to *ask* Stewart if I can see Matt.

What will this mean for you, Molly?

Here is a clue. I want to *inform* Stew of my plans.

I write, *9 is great. Let me know the spot and I'll be there.*

Suddenly, the day stretching before me doesn't seem so bleak. Another clue. I scoop Nate out of the tub and wrap him in a hooded towel. I make airplane sounds as I whoosh him into the kids' room, where Daniel is intently filling in a SpongeBob sticker book.

"Which underwear do you want today?" I say to Nate. "SpongeBob or Diego?"

Nate glances at Daniel's book. "SpongeBob!"

"I'll find them," Daniel says, standing up to assume the big brother role. As the two of them rummage through the closet, I knock on Stewart's studio door.

"Hey," I say. "Matt wants to get a drink tonight. I said I'd meet him at nine. Cool?"

Stew swivels his chair to face me. "Very cool," he says, raising one eyebrow.

"Cool," I say again stupidly. "I'm going to take the kids to the playground."

"Have fun," he says, his eyebrow still lifted.

I go through the motions of the rest of my day, relying on autonomic responses. At the playground, I obey my children's commands to *Look at me!* as they go down the twisty slide, attempt the monkey bars, walk across the spiderweb ropes. I look, I smile, I clap. I push them on the swings. I procure snacks when hunger is expressed. I am ready with a wardrobe change when the juice box is spilled. When we get home, my hands know how to make rocket-ship ravioli, how to steam broccoli, where the toys go. Stew emerges from his studio around seven o'clock, and I sneak in a shower. I get both boys into bed by a miraculous 8:05 p.m. And when Stewart and I sit across from each other at the kitchen table, unwrapping chopsticks, eating sushi and edamame, I stay fixed on each task. It isn't until I've cleared the plates and am standing at the sink that Stewart creeps up behind me, grabs me around the middle, kisses my ear.

"Ready for your big date?" he whispers.

"It's just drinks," I say. I will myself to sound casual, but I'm sure Stewart can feel my quickened pulse. "He lives with his girl-friend, remember?"

"I know." He moves his kisses down the side of my neck. "Can you feel how turned on I am?" He pushes his hardness against my backside.

"Yes," I say. But I want to step away. I want to think about Matt, not Stewart. The reminder of Stewart's pleasure feels like an intrusion.

What will this mean for you, Molly?

This is about *my* desire, not Stewart's.

I push the thought away and turn around to face Stew. I force a smile and kiss him lightly on the lips.

"I have to get going. I'll text you later."

THUNDER IS RUMBLING BY the time I reach the block where I'm supposed to meet Matt. It's one of those South Slope bars that's too hip for signage. I walk past it twice, panicking and wishing I'd brought an umbrella, before I realize I've found it. Inside, I scan the barstools, expecting to see him perched on one. Instead, my eyes find him at a small table in the corner. He looks uncomfortable, like a long-legged bird in a stolen nest. He smiles, and I muster a weak wave.

I walk over and bend to hug him just as he stands to hug me.

We meet somewhere in the middle, our jaws colliding. Instead of laughing, which would signal this moment as light comedy, I pull back in awkward silence. Matt bolts for the bar, mumbling, "Let me get you a drink."

I take off my jacket, adjust my sleeves, hang my bag on the back of the chair. I close my eyes and take deep breaths. I wish I'd had a beer before I left the house.

I hear Matt's footsteps approaching the table and arrange my face into a mask of tranquility. He sets our pint glasses down, and then, abandoning the chair across the table where his jacket still remains, he sits next to me.

I feel his knee against mine—a feeling I've craved for weeks—and there is no mistaking our intentions this time. I slurp at my beer and avoid his gaze until I can't. We stare at each other for a long beat. Then he breaks into a smile.

"Hi there, Molly," he says, the laughter back in his eyes. I'm so grateful for that laughter.

"Hi there, Matt."

Conversation skates along the surface, but nothing can keep my attention off the pressure of Matt's knee against mine. Even when he stands to go to the bar for our next round, we settle back into our seats with our legs drawn to the same position, like the alphabet magnets Daniel likes to hold a millimeter from the refrigerator, just to feel them pulled from his hand.

And then he says it.

"Do you want to come over?"

"What?" I say. But I've anticipated these words since the night I met him. I've imagined them without believing they'd be said, without knowing what I'd say if and when the moment of deciding ever arrived.

He swipes his hand down his face, as if to clear the cobwebs of uncertainty. He looks at me.

"My girlfriend is out of town," he says. "I live close by."

So this is why he wanted to meet not at the Gate, but someplace nearer his apartment. He probably awakened early, helped her carry her suitcase to a waiting taxi, and then hurried back inside to send me a text and invite me out. He's come as close to asking me to sleep with him as he can get without being completely overt.

Matt continues, trying to fill the silence I've created. "I'd really like you to come over."

My reply feels more like an inevitability than a choice.

"Okay."

Outside, the rain has started coming down in metallic sheets. Matt takes off his jacket and holds it over my head as we run down the slick sidewalk, the drumbeat of the rain merging with the drumming of my heart, urging me on. We are there in only a minute or two, but he is already soaked, his shirt clinging to his skin as he unlocks the door, opens it, follows me inside.

And here we are, facing each other in his kitchen.

WHEN I FIND MYSELF out in the storm once again, all I can think to do is text Stewart. He is the only one who can make this okay. Because it's real now, not a hypothetical scenario, a fantasy woven in our marital bed.

Should I go back? I've written, huddled under an awning, oblivious to the flashes of lightning closing in. I stare at the phone, willing it to answer me, and within seconds it does.

For such an enormous question, Stewart's answer is brief.

Go for it.

Go for it. Not within the safety of our marriage—*go for something outside of it.* And although I've received Stew's blessing, even his encouragement, I am not doing this for my husband. I am not doing this to keep the excitement in our marriage alive. I am racing back to another man's apartment because it is what *I* want. I am climbing his stairs and ringing the bell and unbuttoning my soaking-wet dress before he even answers the door because I want *him*.

IT'S AFTER THREE A.M. when I leave Matt's apartment. I'm back on the puddle-soaked sidewalk, which looks different to me now. The storm is over; calm is restored. I walk toward home, my dress and shoes still damp, and I pass the awning where I'd stopped to text Stewart just a few hours before.

At home, I strip off my wet clothes in the laundry room, grab a T-shirt from the floor, and put it on. I climb into bed, hoping that Stewart is asleep, but then I hear his voice in the darkness.

"So how was it, my sexy wife?"

A siren of warning goes off within my depths, and I give incomplete information.

"It was fun," I say.

I do not say that all I want is to go back, to feel Matt's hands on my body, another man's mouth on my own.

CHAPTER 4

NATE WAKES UP EARLY the next morning, saving me from my thoughts. I've barely slept, but I'm not tired. A manic energy transports me as I carry Nate into the kitchen, blowing raspberries on his cheeks while he giggles. I pour Cheerios into a bowl as my mind continues to buzz, blurring every action into the background. There's no use fighting it.

I bring Nate and his Cheerios into the living room and plunk him down in front of the television.

"Noggin," says a cheerful voice. "It's like preschool on TV!"

Nate watches Moose and his mute bird friend, Zee, introduce the next show as I stretch out on the couch behind him and close my eyes. I fidget with my wedding ring as I treat myself to a private screening of images from last night. I don't want to lose a single frame.

Matt opens the door. I've already unbuttoned my dress to my belly button, and I watch his eyes hover between my face and my chest. My bra has a front clasp, and I undo it there in the doorway. Me. The girl who couldn't make eye contact with boys in high school, the girl who lost her virginity when she was almost nineteen and got dumped the next day. I am not this girl anymore. I am sexy, confident. I fall forward into his waiting body, our mouths connecting as one of his hands cups my breast and the other presses into the back of my head, fingers woven with hair. I feel the smoothness of his clean-shaven face. He pulls me inside and kicks the door shut. We stumble past the kitchen, where we'd kissed just ten minutes ago, where I'd backed away from him as if he were a poisonous thing—but that was the girl I used to be. Now I find myself gulping him down, and discover that he is not poison at all, but a drug I need in order to survive, in order to keep that other sad and careful girl in her rightful place, under the cellar stairs, quiet as a mouse. We topple onto his bed. I reach for his belt while keeping my mouth attached to his, tasting the drug on his tongue and drinking deeply . . .

"Mommy?" I open my eyes and see Nate's little face, inches from my own. Behind him, Dora the Explorer has convinced Tico the Squirrel to give her a ride over the bridge. But the Grumpy Old Troll is making trouble.

"I ate all my Cheerios. Can I have some more, please?"

"Of course, sweetie. Just give me one minute."

"Okay." He reaches out a chubby hand and rests it on my arm, then twists his body to watch Dora solve her next crisis.

I close my eyes again and try to resume where I left off. *I unbuckle his belt, unbutton his jeans, slide my hand inside his underwear and feel the size, the shape of his hard cock . . .* A kiss on my cheek, the scrape of stubble. I see Stewart's face now, upside down above me, his nose twitching.

"You smell different," he says. "Did you shower when you got home last night?"

"Sorry," I say. "It was really late. I didn't think you'd mind."

"Well, I kinda do," he says, and walks away.

What will this mean for you, Molly?

I don't know what it means, and I don't want to know. The danger I've suspected all along is palpable now. I am both the character in a horror movie, entering the darkened woods where the killer hides, and the anxious spectator in the theater, wanting to yell, *Don't go in there!* But everyone knows what happens next. It's part of the thrill.

I pull out my phone and type a text:

Sorry, Mitchell. I need to cancel our appointment next week.

I PLAN A TRIP with Daniel and Nate to see my parents. My mother's balance is getting worse, and this visit is overdue. But there's another reason I want to see her, a conversation I want to have—or, more accurately, a conversation I want to finish.

Stewart has to work, of course, and is staying home. The night before we leave, I'm up late packing—a suitcase full of clothes for myself and the boys, two carry-on bags with toys and snacks for the plane ride. Stew wanders into the room and moves a pile of underwear. He sits on the bed.

"Can I talk to you for a minute?"

"Sure," I say, not looking up. "Do you know where Nate's rain boots are?" The weather forecast for Chicago is dreary, but I'm determined to get the kids outside.

"No idea," he says. "So Lena invited me over this weekend. While you guys are away."

I stop folding shirts and look at him. "Lena? As in, your ex-girlfriend Lena?"

"Yeah," says Stewart. "I think I told you before—she's going through a pretty rough divorce. She just wants to talk."

"Just talking, huh?" I drop my eyes and pretend to study the piles of clothing again.

"I think so. But what if it weren't just talking? How would you feel about that?"

My heart squeezes into a tiny ball, wedging itself against my lungs and stopping my breath. Of all the girlfriends from Stew's past, Lena is one of a select few who broke up with *him* rather than the other way around. But Stewart remained friends with her—Lena was one of five ex-girlfriends who attended our wedding, which has to be some sort of record. I'm not exactly jealous of Lena. She's older than I am and has changed over the years into a matronly type. But I know that in a corner of Stew's brain, he wants to show Lena what she missed. And the thought of them together makes me feel like I've fallen to the bottom of a well.

"I'm not sure," I say, still not looking at him. I'm afraid I'll start to cry if I do. The tears have been close to the surface ever since my night with Matt. Or, more accurately, after a few days passed and I realized I might never see him again. His girlfriend is back, and he's awash with guilt. "I guess it's okay. I mean, it's not fair if I'm the only one who gets to . . . you know . . ."

"Cool," says Stew, standing to go. "I doubt anything's going to happen. She's still pretty hung up on her husband, but I wanted to make sure you're all right with it. Just in case."

"Uh-huh," I say. "I get it."

Stewart pauses in the doorway. "Are you sure it's okay?"

"Yup." I finally look up and give him a tight smile. Doesn't he know I'm lying? "I'm just a little stressed about packing."

"I'll drive you to the airport in the morning," he says. "I'm going to miss you guys."

Why would you miss us? I think. *You're going to have an empty house and a hot date with Lena.*

"We'll miss you, too," I say.

BY THE TIME THE plane lands at O'Hare, I have a migraine. My father has offered to pick us up at the airport, and I'm relieved to see him, hands clasped behind his back—an upright sentinel— near our baggage claim carousel. His salt-and-pepper beard is neatly trimmed, but his eyebrows point in multiple directions. He scans the crowd and I wave until he sees me.

"Hoppin!" Nate screams, using the name given to my father by my oldest nephew. He crashes into my father's legs, and my dad grunts as if he's been hit by a linebacker, much to Nate's delight. My dad tousles Nate's hair and extends a hand to shake Daniel's.

Really? I think. *He's only eight years old and we've abandoned hugs? I guess I should be grateful he doesn't make his grandkids call him Phil.*

"Hi, Dad," I say, wrapping him in an embrace before he can deflect it.

"Hi, kiddo." His arms dangle awkwardly behind me, but he manages a few pats on my back.

In the car, I quiz my dad on my mother's health. "How is she doing? Really?"

"Oh, we're both hanging in there," he says, his eyes on the road. "I've taken over certain things, like the laundry. Stairs are hard for her, you know. And I'm doing most of the shopping and cooking."

He glances over at me, gauging my reaction to this development. When I was growing up, my father never did much of the housework, and I know he wants me to congratulate him now. I give him a minimal nod, a half-hearted raise of the eyebrows. But it feels like too little, too late. I think about my mother struggling on the stairs. I'm silent as I take it all in.

The migraine stays with me. As I hug my mother hello. As I follow Nate around the house, warning him not to torment the dog. As I drink coffee, as I make lunch, as I watch the boys climb the jungle gym or push them on the swings at the drizzly playground, the migraine is my constant companion, thudding in the background to crowd out thoughts of Stewart and Lena. Before I get into bed at night, I swallow Tylenol PM, which I hide from my mother.

I have a few minutes before the pills take effect, minutes during which I lose myself in the blue patterned wallpaper. For most of my childhood, this was my parents' room. I didn't inherit it until the summer before eleventh grade, after my sister left home and my parents renovated her bedroom into a master suite for themselves. But I never made the room my own. The rug, the lamp, the dresser, even the bed itself—it all once belonged to my parents. And it all still feels like it's theirs.

I try not to think of who else might have lain here. But it's hard not to remember what I know.

ABOUT A YEAR BEFORE Daniel was born, Stewart and I drove up to Boston for the weekend. My favorite aunt, my mother's older sister Anne, was visiting her son, my cousin Henry, to celebrate her sixtieth birthday. Anne was the wild child to my goody-two-shoes mother. She was divorced and drank too much and had just gotten a tattoo. Anne treated us all to dinner, and at some point during our surf-and-turf combo meal, after the third vodka tonic had been served, the topic turned to family. It was rare for me to see Anne without my mother present. I took advantage and confided.

"You know what drives me crazy about my mom?" I said. "She's always so damn perfect. It's hard to ever get angry at her."

"Hmph," Anne snorted. "Your mother's not so perfect."

"What do you mean?"

"Oh, I shouldn't have said anything," Anne replied, clearly enjoying my confusion. I noticed that Henry was now intently drinking water, avoiding my gaze.

"What?" I asked again. "Tell me."

Anne straightened herself up and took a leisurely swig. And then: "She had an affair."

"What?!" The tables around us seemed to disappear, and a spotlight descended on Anne and the slim, cylindrical glass that she brought to her lips again. "When? Who was it?"

Stewart put his hand on my leg.

"It's not a big deal, baby," he said. "Your parents are still married. And they seem to love each other."

"It's a big deal to me," I said. I thought I knew my mother. I thought she was one kind of person, and now I was being told she was someone else. A dissembler. A liar. "Come on, Anne. Who was it?"

Anne looked directly at me. "I think you already know."

I did know. Jim.

Jim was my mother's best friend. He was eight years younger—the exact same age difference that exists between Matt and me. Jim was silly and lively and could do funny voices. They met when he was fresh out of college and subbing at the high school where my mother taught English. Like my mom, he was a spiritual seeker by nature. When I was six, he brought my mom to a Mahikari dojo, a place where members of a Japanese healing practice could exchange "divine light." Eventually, my mother and Jim made a trip to L.A. together. They took a weeklong course and became Mahikari members.

I can still picture the two of them exchanging light in the living room. My dad stayed out late on nights when Jim came over, and my sister locked herself in her room. But I didn't like being alone. I sat on the stairs and peeked down at them while they took turns giving and receiving light. The whole thing took a long time, filling the two hours between dinner and my bedtime. Even though I had to be quiet, I was glad Jim was there; otherwise, my mother would want to give me light instead.

First, my mother gave and Jim received. They faced each other, sitting with their legs tucked underneath them. My mother did the chant, which I already knew by heart. Then, for ten minutes, she held her hand above Jim's forehead, sliding one hand to take the place of the other when her arm got tired. If they did an extended session, Jim then lay on his belly—twenty minutes of light on various spots up and down his spine. Touching was minimal. Sometimes she probed a thumb into his flesh to feel for toxins. When she found one, her hand rose again, two inches above his body, and the invisible light poured from her palm. When they did this, Jim was very serious. It made me uncomfortable, like he'd turned into a different person.

On the nights when Jim didn't come over, my mother usually talked to him on the phone. I could always tell who she was talking to because of the sounds she made. First she shrieked with laughter. Then there was silence as she fell back in her chair, paralyzed, followed by desperate gasps for air. I knew what Jim was doing on the other end of the line. He did the same thing when he joined us for dinner at the kitchen table, before the exchange of light. He'd start by saying something mildly funny—to my mom, at least—and when she gave a little chuckle, he went deadpan, his voice a parody of sternness: "Mary, that's not funny. Stop laughing, Mary."

That's all it took. He was the only one who made my mother laugh like that.

I loved hearing her laugh, my mother, who was always busy performing some duty—making dinner, washing dishes, grading papers at the kitchen table late into the night. Or exchanging light with Jim. There was no time in her life for more than these obligations.

But in her laughter with Jim, I heard something else. Something lighter and free.

———

FOR THE NEXT YEAR, throughout my pregnancy, I held on to the secret Anne had revealed. But when Daniel was just a few days old, Stewart's father got sick. A week later, he was in the hospital with a serious case of pneumonia. Stewart had to leave his newborn son to be at the bedside of his dying father.

Everything was confusion, and I was grateful to have the singular task of caring for my baby. Motherhood wrapped me in a protective shroud. My tender breasts were Daniel's only source of food, and I spent hours and hours of my days and nights nursing him. My mother came to help, to take care of *her* baby, she told me, while I cared for mine.

Daniel was attached to a breast most of the time, leaving me desperately thirsty. My mother brought me plastic cups of ice water with a long straw for hands-free drinking, then sat on the couch beside me as I nursed. Our conversations ranged from the micro—the best salve for my sore nipples, burping methods for Daniel—to the macro, the questions of life and death that hovered all around us.

On the day Stewart called to tell me his father had died, I put the phone down and leaned against my mother, crying onto her shoulder as Daniel continued his endless suckling. Exhausted and overwhelmed, I couldn't hold my question any longer. It slipped from my grasp, landing on the sliver of couch between us.

"I know about your affair," I said. "It's none of my business, but I want to ask one thing. Does Dad know?"

My mom was quiet for a moment, looking at her hands in her lap. I looked at them, too. Her mysterious symptoms had just begun, and the fingers of her left hand wouldn't straighten anymore. They curled around an invisible egg.

"It was your father's idea," she replied.

———

WHEN THE TYLENOL PM kicks in, I fall into fitful dreams in which I go back to our Brooklyn home or meet Stewart at his office, a restaurant—the scenario keeps changing—only to find that another woman is already there with him, taking my place. Five or six hours later, when Nate drags me from my sleep, I pop two caffeinated Excedrin. But the migraine thuds on.

By the last night at my parents' house, I'm not sure if the headache is lifting or if I've just gotten used to it. I tuck Daniel and Nate into the bunk beds that now occupy my old room, the one that was mine as a little kid, with the butterfly wallpaper I'd once chosen. Then I knock on my parents' bathroom door.

My mother's voice answers, forever cheerful, regardless of what is happening: "Come in!"

I find her seated on the toilet, wrestling with her compression socks. A few years ago, while grading her students' *Siddhartha* essays, just as I finished my first year as an English teacher, my mother discovered she could no longer control the pen in her hand. Her left big toe started to drag. Over time, her words became jumbled as they left her mouth, and her balance worsened. She went to the Mayo Clinic in Minnesota, but the doctors remained stumped. *Ataxia,* my mother continues to call it, in lieu of a real diagnosis. During a visit after Nate was born, we'd brainstormed possible causes. *Maybe it's all my repressed rage,* she'd mused. As a mother of two, I'd understood exactly what she meant. Sometimes I didn't know what was more likely to destroy me: the rage itself or my efforts to stifle it. But now I wonder, is her rage even deeper than I imagined?

"Hi, Mom," I say. "Do you need some help?" Getting dressed and undressed seems to take all my mother's time these days.

"Nope! This is my physical therapy. Did the kids go down okay?"

"We'll find out." I sit down on the bathroom floor and lean against the smoothness of the tub. I look at my mother's face, still pretty in everyone's opinion but her own, her brow furrowed in concentration. It's hard to tell if she's trying to put the sock on or take it off.

"I'm so glad you're here," she says, the sock hanging off her toes. "We haven't had a real chance to talk. Tell me everything. How's Stewart?"

Tell me everything. About the other man you slept with? About the woman Stewart may be fucking this very instant?

Your mother's not so perfect, Anne had said to me. It turns out I'm not so perfect, either.

"He's fine," I say, "but sometimes it's hard. With the kids and everything, you know?" I look at her again, hoping to convey with my eyes all the things I can't say.

"A married couple is like two stones in a river," she says. The sock is off now. She focuses on lowering her foot to the floor and then turns her full attention to me. "You spend your life rubbing up against each other, creating friction. But that's how you smooth out each other's rough edges."

I swallow my rising tears as she continues to look at me. She sees. She knows.

"Stewart is your other river stone, honey. I've never had any doubt about that."

I nod, then look away. I want to ask so many things. About my father. About her rage. About what it means and doesn't mean to be a wife, to be a mother. But the words won't come. And then the migraine rushes back in, gripping the part of my mind that might have formulated a question.

"I'm exhausted," I say instead, standing to kiss her on the top of her head. "Good night, Mom. I love you."

Lying in my parents' old bed, thinking about Stewart and Lena, I want to go back to the bathroom, where my mother is still likely to be, painstakingly brushing her teeth or washing her face. She is so slow now that her bedtime routine takes over an hour to complete. But I can't make myself do it. Aside from that one conversation, in the wake of Daniel's birth and the death of Stewart's father, my mother and I have never spoken openly about sex. And even though she had my dad's explicit permission, she still called her relationship with Jim an "affair." I could hear the shame in her voice when she told me, as if the encouragement of your husband hardly mattered. As if nothing really excused a woman's desire for anything or anyone outside the confines of marriage.

But is my mother's shame the reason I won't ask her my questions? The reason I don't want to find out if my father had "affairs," too? If my mother was also crushed with the jealousy and pain I feel at the thought of Stewart sleeping with Lena?

I don't want to ask because I don't want to tell her about myself, I realize. I don't want my mother to know the truth about my own marriage. Because I'm wondering if I've made a horrible mistake.

Because for reasons I can't articulate, I'm ashamed, too.

THE NEXT DAY, MY head still pounding, our plane touches down at LaGuardia. Stewart picks us up at baggage claim. Nate and Daniel throw themselves at him. He holds them tight, leaning over their heads to kiss me.

"I have a bad headache," I tell him.

"Sorry, baby. Let's get you home." I watch how he picks up Nate with one arm, how he reaches to the carousel and lifts our heavy suitcase with the other. His broad shoulders, his biceps swelling beneath his T-shirt, his facial scruff flecked with red and gold.

I follow Stew and the boys to the parking garage, watching his confident walk, his cute butt, his fun, affectionate manner with our sons. Panic wells up within me. My husband is sexy, a great dad, a total catch. How had I forgotten?

The boys keep up a constant chatter the whole ride home, and I close my eyes, feel the pain throbbing behind my thoughts. Soon Stewart and I will be alone, and I'll no longer wonder. I'll no longer have a way out of this dread, the hope that *maybe they didn't* to slump my weight against in relief.

When we get inside the house, Daniel runs to his room and Nate goes in search of the cat. Stewart carries our suitcase up the stairs and I trail him with leaden legs, an automaton on a mission that will end in self-destruction.

In our room, I close the door behind myself.

"You want this on the bed?" Stew asks, gesturing to the suitcase.

I stand mute, my knees shaking. Spots float in my field of vision. My voice emerges in a whisper.

"Did you sleep with her?"

Stew drops his head along with the suitcase and lets out a deep sigh. He looks at me, and I see the answer in his eyes before he says it.

"Yes."

My legs give way. I crumple onto the floor next to the bed. I'm afraid I might vomit.

"Molly . . . ," he begins.

But I can hardly hear him. I'm at the bottom of the well now. From far away, words and phrases assemble themselves without sense or connection. *She doesn't mean anything to me. . . . You told me it was okay. . . . Why are you reacting like this?*

Only one syllable from his mouth reaches me. That *yes.*

Yes, I hear, *everything you feared is happening.*

I WAKE UP IN a dark room. My head now feels bruised rather than shattered. I get out of bed and pad down the stairs. The house is quiet. Stewart is in the kitchen, washing dishes with his earphones in.

I creep up behind him and wrap my arms around his middle, resting my face on his back. He turns off the faucet, wipes his hands on his jeans, pulls out one earpiece.

"You put the kids to bed," I say. "Thank you."

"Of course," he answers, not turning around. His voice is wooden.

"I'm sorry," I say.

"What for?" he asks. Stewart hates it when I apologize without knowing why. I think about how many times my mother said *I'm sorry* over the weekend, and for years before that, throughout my entire life, in fact. She apologized constantly. For nothing. For everything.

"I don't know."

We stand in silence for a while, my hands gripping his chest. I start to cry.

"I'm getting your shirt wet," I say.

He turns around. "Let's talk."

We go into the living room and sit down on the couch. It's nice to feel his body next to mine without having to look directly at him. I wish I could crawl into his lap. But there's an armor around him, an invisible force field I can't penetrate.

"I don't know how to talk to you about this," he says, looking at his hands. "I don't want to feel guilty about doing something you gave me permission to do."

He's angry at me, I realize. *He* is angry at *me*. My head clouds over and the urge to vomit returns.

"I don't think I should have told you about Lena," he continues. "I'm into hearing about you and Matt, but I know you don't feel the same way about me being with another woman."

He's right, of course, but hearing about it is the least of my concerns. The problem is the fact that it's happening at all. I think back to my mother: *It was your father's idea.* But this is different. Sleeping with Matt was *my* idea, right?

"Lena is never going to replace you, Molly." He glances at me before returning his gaze to his hands. "She's my friend, but that's it. Just like you and Matt. It doesn't mean anything."

I can't breathe, and dizzy nausea waves over me. *What will this mean for you, Molly?* I'm still not sure what sex with Matt means to me, but it's not friendship.

Stewart keeps talking, either oblivious or willfully ignoring my silence. "But I'll admit. It feels good to be seen as attractive, y'know?"

Of course I know. It's the same way for me. But I'd forgotten that Stewart needs reassurances, too. On an early date, Stew and I had visited his parents' home on Long Island. He'd shown me a picture taken at his bar mitzvah: a fat kid stuffed into a cream-colored suit, his jacket straining at the buttons, thick glasses, acne, curly hair the color of a new penny (a "Jewfro," Stew called it), sandwiched between his smiling parents and his tall, slim older brother. "My mom calls my brother 'the good-looking one,'" Stew had told me, and I'd gasped in horror.

Tears start to fall again. I think of how I'd seen him in the airport that afternoon. I don't know how long it's been since I told him he was sexy. He tells me all the time, but I still don't believe him. Why can't we give that to each other? What is wrong with us?

He picks up my hand—a limp, dead thing—and holds it in his. "I think we have a decision to make. Do you want to stop?"

Of course I do. We have to stop. I can't share Stewart. I can't share him with Lena, the woman who wishes she were his wife, the woman who has known him longer than I have, the woman whose children call him Uncle Stew.

But at the same time, I can't *not* see Matt again. I still can't explain why. Maybe it's like Stewart said, about being seen with fresh eyes. About feeling not like a wife or a mom but a desirable woman again. Maybe my feelings for Matt are nothing more than an addiction to how I feel when I'm with him: shiny and new.

"I don't know," I say to Stew.

"Do you want me to do a puppet show?" I look up. "Talk to me," he says in a goofy voice, his left hand speaking to his right.

I want so badly to give in to his silliness. Stewart's ability to make me laugh, even in the midst of shit shows and dumpster fires, is his superpower, high on the list of reasons I married him. But now I'm questioning his motives. Is he just trying to distract me from the chasm beneath us? *Watch the puppet show; don't look down.*

It's too exhausting. I decide to trust him because I don't see any other way. I throw my arms around his neck.

"I love you so much," I say.

"I love you too, my baby," he answers. "I will always love you. But let's try out a new rule for a while. I'm not going to tell you any more about what I'm doing."

"Okay," I say, my head pulsing like a strobe light, turning my thoughts formless, impossible to examine.

"But you," he says with a devilish smile, "have to tell me everything."

———

THAT NIGHT, I LIE in bed, spooned into Stewart.

I can't remove an image from my brain, one from over ten years ago, when I traveled to Venezuela with my friend Maria, a trip that coincided with Stewart's and my first wedding anniversary. It was symbolic, I thought, that we didn't need to be together on that day, that although we were married, we could still have our own independent lives.

One weekend, Maria and I went on a white-water rafting trip. On the second day, our guides stopped at a bridge. It was a popular spot for people to jump into the river and let the rapids carry them a bit, after which they'd swim at a right angle to reach the shore. Apparently, there were people who found this fun.

I, however, am deathly afraid of heights. But an impulse overcame me. Here was an opportunity to challenge my fear, to not be the cautious one for once, to be bold. I volunteered to jump first. Maria later described the scene from her perspective.

"It was like watching someone attempt suicide," she said.

I ignored all the advice the guides had given—*Be sure to point your toes, cross your arms over your chest, jump several feet out.* Instead, I simply stepped off the bridge, limbs flailing, and landed in the water with a smack. Stunned, I began to drift, not making any attempt to move my arms or legs. Maria jumped into the water after me and dragged my useless body with her to the riverbank.

"Don't ever do that again!" she yelled at me.

"Okay," I said, returning to my docile self as she kept me afloat. "I won't."

Later, I developed a bruise over my hip and thigh where my flesh had struck the water's surface. It was the diameter of a Frisbee, green and purple and gold, and Maria took a photo of it to remind me of my promise. But the bruise has healed, the photo is lost, and I know I will break my pledge.

I am about to make another insane leap.

CHAPTER 5

OVER THE NEXT FOUR years, I sleep with Matt only a handful of times—when his girlfriend is out of town or when Stewart is at a conference and the kids are at summer camp. The pattern goes something like this: After we have sex, Matt texts me to say he can't do this anymore. He feels too guilty. I cry and mope about, battling migraines more days than not, and then bury myself in motherly duties. My children are still young. They need me. This is all for the best, I tell myself. Then, after a couple of months pass, Matt and I start texting again—every week or two, then more frequently, our messages marked by fraudulent chastity as anticipation builds toward an opportunity to see each other. His girlfriend has a work trip. Or I will have the house to myself. Most importantly, we never plan to sleep together. We simply *check in,* see if the other is free to go out for a drink, to talk.

I hide the fact that Stew knows about these liaisons. I want Matt to think the two of us are sinking in identical boats, that he and I are grappling with the same demons. But in truth, the closer we get to these "innocent" dates, the lighter I feel, the less frequently my migraines occur. When I know I'll see Matt soon, I'm more patient with the kids, more eager to have sex with Stewart.

On the nights Matt and I meet—and it's always at night—electricity courses through my body the moment his green eyes meet mine. We spend an hour or two on our best behavior, drinking steadily to dismantle any pesky inhibitions, until finally, our knees touch under the table and we keep them there. Our eyes lock, we drunkenly stumble to his apartment or my house, whichever is vacant, and we strip each other naked, fuck furiously but always briefly, and have perhaps ten minutes of strained pillow talk before Matt's guilt and my shame rear their ugly heads once again. And the cycle repeats.

Matt's guilt makes sense to me, but my shame is less clear. I've excused away any responsibility for Matt's girlfriend. *(If he's cheating on her before they're even married, their relationship must be doomed, right?)* And I have my husband's permission. Nevertheless, there is something about acknowledging my own unmet needs that makes me look away.

In bed with Stew, however, my shame disappears and Matt belongs to my marriage again, a prop, as he was always intended to be. Even semiannual interludes with Matt can keep me in a froth. *Do you want to see how I sucked Matt's cock? Do you want me to show you how I rode him?* I release all my fear, all my desire onto Stewart. Our sex feels dangerous, as if we're leaning over an abyss, grabbing each other tightly so as not to fall in. Sometimes, when Stewart does something new—moves his tongue differently, puts my leg over one shoulder in an unfamiliar pose—I freeze. *Where did he learn to do that?* I wonder. But I don't dare ask. I shake my head back and forth to kill the question, like a dog with a rat in its mouth, and will myself into a primal state, my mind free from thought. Then I orgasm more powerfully than I did even in the early days of our marriage.

I DON'T KNOW HOW often Stewart is seeing Lena. But I do know it's happening. One day, while doing laundry, I reach into Stew's pockets to clear out the tissues and gum wrappers, the receipts and dry-cleaning tickets. I feel what seems to be a credit card. I pull it out, a piece of rectangular plastic. I stare for several seconds before I make sense of what I see.

Hilton. Enjoy your stay.

It's a hotel key card, and it's speaking to me in Stewart's voice.

I'm not going to tell you any more about what I'm doing, it says. *Instead, I'll leave hotel keys in my pocket. I know you do all the laundry. You're sure to find it. This way, you can picture us in a hotel room together. If you recall which jeans I wore on which day, you might even be able to figure out the exact night it happened. You'll think back to that text, when I told you I was working late. You'll remember that was the night I came home at four thirty in the morning and kissed you while you were sleeping, kissed you with the mouth that kissed hers, that had roamed over her entire body, perhaps, that had made her moan and cry out.*

I think about all the years I've spent my nights alone with the kids—the dinners, the bedtimes, the dishes, the loneliness of doing it all by myself—because Stew had to work. I check in with my sense of reality. *Was he truly at the office all those times?* Yes, I believe he was. After all, he's clearly a bad liar, one who can't manage to cover his tracks now.

But another thought is rising within me, despite my efforts to tamp it down. All of those nights, he could have come home instead. He's blowing off work to be with *her* now, isn't he?

I feel my jealousy mingle with the resentment I've kept at bay for years, every time the feeling of being alone in the epic job of parenting crept along my temples, tightened my throat, bored its way into my bowels. But looking at my anger is like looking at the sun. It hurts to stare at it for too long, making a full examination impossible. And when I look away, everything is colored by fury.

I drop the key card in the trash.

———

IN ALL THIS TIME, I've never invited Matt to our house when the kids were home—until today. Maybe it's that Nate is eight years old now, and I feel confident he won't awaken during the night. Maybe finding the Hilton key prompts this reckless action, as if I've knocked back a potent jealousy-anger cocktail, clouding my judgment. I find that my resentment is directed less at Lena and more at Stewart's freedom to do as he pleases, to go to hotels without worrying about details such as bedtimes or babysitters. Anyway, I rationalize, Daniel and Nate are upstairs, asleep in their beds. And we're two floors away, down in the guest room with a door that locks, an available escape route under the stoop.

Clothes litter the floor, and I tell Matt I have to check on the kids. I leave him lying on the bed and run naked up the stairs to the kitchen—beyond reckless, really. I don't check on the kids at all. Instead, I text Stewart. He agreed so readily to stay late at the office, facilitating this wild scheme, that I've started to feel guilty.

Matt's still here, I write. *But don't worry. He has nothing on you as a lover.*

I mean this, and I don't mean it. Sex is different with Matt, exciting in its illicit nature. But Stew knows my body so well. It would take years for Matt to catch up. Mostly, I want to reassure Stewart, to tell him a palatable version of "everything I'm doing" as he has requested.

I hit Send. And see that I've sent my message to the wrong man.

This time I do text Stew. *How do I unsend a message??* I write frantically. *I thought I was sending a text to you but I sent it to Matt!*

Stewart tries to help, but it's no use. The text remains sent. I run back downstairs—still naked—and make chaotic small talk as I rifle through our discarded clothes, looking for Matt's phone like it's a time bomb. I need to delete that message.

"Molly," Matt says to me. I don't look up.

"Molly," he repeats. "Who was that text for?"

He is still lying on the bed but has put on his jeans. He's holding his phone, which must have been in his back pocket.

I stare at the phone in his hand, trying to figure out if there's any way I can still lie. There isn't.

"It was for Stewart," I say. "But I didn't mean it. You're an amazing lover. I was just trying to make him feel better."

"That's the least of my worries, Molly. He knows I'm here?"

I nod. I see something new in his eyes when he looks at me. Disgust, maybe—whether it's disgust for me, for himself, or both of us, I can't say. My throat dries up, as if I've swallowed sawdust. I'm unable to produce sound.

"I gotta go," he says, shaking his head. "I have to think."

I watch in silence as he stuffs his feet into his shoes and pulls his shirt over his head. He is out the door so quickly I can't be sure he was ever here at all. I send one more text to Stew: *He left. Can you come home please?*

I cannot bear to look at the sheets, tousled by what will surely be the last time I ever feel his body against mine. But I force myself to strip the bed, to throw the sheets into the washing machine, to take a shower and put on pajamas.

When Stewart comes home, he holds me and tells me not to worry.

"It's not such a big deal," Stew says. "Why should he care?"

I can't explain how I know, but I'm certain this is the end. The way he looked at me. Like I've been using him all along. And maybe I have. But not the way he thinks, not only as a prop in my marriage, like I've wanted Stewart to believe. No, I've been using Matt as a portal to another world, a world where I can run naked to my own kitchen without feeling like I'm doing something wrong. But that world isn't real. And the portal has closed.

I lie awake for hours, and as soon as the first bar of light appears in the bedroom window, I text Matt, trying to explain. He writes a terse reply.

I wish you all the best, Molly, but I'm done. Good-bye.

I sleepwalk through the rest of the day, numbed by the shock of what has happened, by the idiocy of my mistake. I've found myself starring in a daytime drama. Lying to Matt for years about Stewart knowing the truth. Having sex in the guest room while my children were asleep upstairs. Traipsing naked through the house. Sending the worst possible text at the worst possible moment to the worst possible person. If these actions weren't mine, the situation would almost be funny. But none of this is someone else's doing. It's all my own. And I'm steeped in shame.

That night, Stewart comes home early. He sees that I'm somewhere else, somewhere he can't reach, and he handles me with care.

"Do you want to talk about it?" he asks after the kids are in bed. I'm lying mute on the couch, my eyes red and swollen.

"I don't know if I can do this anymore," I say.

He nods silently. And then: "Do you want me to stop seeing Lena?"

His words feel like a lifesaving buoy. I rise up from the depths to grab hold of it.

"You would do that for me?" I ask.

"Of course," he says. "You're more important to me than anyone else in the world. Let's take a break. Until you're feeling better."

The buoy deflates a bit, and I sink below the surface once more. A break. Not the end.

"You don't get it," I say. "I don't think I'm *ever* going to be able to do this again. It hurts too much." I don't even know how to sort out all the hurt. It hurts to share Stewart, and it hurts to lose Matt. But it also hurts to think that this part of my life is over. That I'll never have the feeling of being shiny and new to someone ever again. That I'll never again be shiny and new to myself.

"I think I *do* get it," Stewart says, taking my hand. "Remember Le Trapeze?"

Of course I remember. Le Trapeze was a seedy sex club we went to before we got married. But if the look in his eye is any indication, we remember it differently. Right now, I'm remembering the two hookers in the ladies' room who talked about their hopes for the evening: that the johns who'd brought them there would take them to McDonald's.

"I didn't like Le Trapeze," I say.

"What? That's not true," he says, waving his hand at me. "If it were, we wouldn't have gone *twice*. There were things you liked, and things you didn't like. It's the same with dating other people."

I have to acknowledge the truth of this. At Le Trapeze, I liked walking around with my breasts exposed. I liked the way Stewart had looked at me, and the way other men had, too. I liked the feeling of breaking out of my good-girl mold, of being daring and desired.

But I didn't like the anonymity of it. I didn't like the feeling of being an interchangeable body. Because of this, I told Stewart I wanted to leave the moment a stranger touched me. And although it was my idea to go back a second time, I got plenty drunk in order to do so.

"I'm not promising anything," I say to Stew. "But I'll think about it. Just give me some time. For starters, I think I need to go back to therapy."

"Great idea," Stewart says, kissing me on the forehead. "As long as I don't have to go."

"SO THE LAST TIME you were here," says Mitchell, "I asked you to think about what it would mean for you to sleep with Matt."

I nod, amazed. It's like we never stopped talking. Even if he reviewed his notes before I walked into the office, there is something genuine in his eyes. I appreciate this feeling Mitchell gives me: of being recognized, remembered, known.

"But last time, I didn't want to think about what it meant. I just wanted to do it." I pause. "And I did sleep with him. A bunch of times." It feels good to confess my sins, and it feels even better that Mitchell doesn't act like I've committed any sins at all.

"And now you sense a change?" he asks. "In terms of being ready to think about it?"

I nod again. "I need to figure some things out," I say. A sudden pain descends on my skull, like a torture device in the shape of a swimming cap. Mitchell notices. I must be wincing.

"What's going on inside you right this moment? Physically, I mean."

"I get headaches," I say. "More like migraines. They can get really bad. But I don't get them all the time."

"Hmm," says Mitchell, making a note. "I think we've just figured out your first bit of homework. Over the next two weeks, I'd like you to write down what you're doing or thinking about whenever you feel a headache coming on."

"Okay," I say, perking up a bit, the torture cap loosening its grip. "I love homework."

"Really?" says Mitchell, laughing. "Why is that?"

I stop to think about it. I remember the day I started third grade, how excited I was, for this was the year when I'd finally get homework.

"I guess because I was good at it?" I say. "On the first day of third grade, I did all my homework for the year—two entire workbooks for reading and math. So I ended up skipping fourth grade."

Mitchell makes another note. I'm not sure how this is relevant to my sex life, or even to my headaches. "You must have been quite young compared to your peers."

"Yeah," I say. "I was already the youngest kid in my grade. So I was only twelve when I started high school. Sixteen when I started college. People used to call me Doogie Howser. But it's not like I was curing cancer or anything. I was just really good at worksheets."

"I'm sure it was more than that," he says with another laugh. I'm glad he finds me so entertaining. "How did you feel about skipping a grade?"

I consider his question. "I liked being thought of as smart," I say. "I liked that the adults thought I was so capable, especially my parents."

Mitchell looks at me, waiting.

"But it was hard being so young." A connection starts to dawn on me. "I was seen as a nerd my whole life. And I never had a boyfriend until my junior year of college. That's the boyfriend I had for four years, right before I met Stewart. William. In fact, that's why Stew said to me—before we were even engaged—that he wanted me to sleep with other people. He thought I missed out on sowing my wild oats or whatever."

I watch Mitchell as he writes something down. "Plus, it turns him on," I say.

Mitchell nods again, still waiting.

"And another thing," I add. "I'm not sure if this is important or not, but my parents had an open marriage, too. They didn't call it that, though. My mother was sleeping with another guy, and my father was the one who encouraged her to do it. Kind of like me and Stewart, actually. But I didn't know about my parents when Stew and I first talked about doing the same thing."

Mitchell raises his eyebrows, and his pen scratches furiously.

By the time our session ends, I'm brimming with homework. First, I must track my headaches. My next assignment, however, is even more important.

"Molly," says Mitchell, first looking at the ceiling to collect his thoughts, then bringing them down to eye level. "You've told me why Stewart thinks you should be in an open marriage. And you've cited your parents' relationship as precedent. But you have yet to articulate what *you* hope to gain from this arrangement. So I'd like for you to keep thinking about that."

I nod, wishing I could bring Mitchell home with me.

"And," he continues, giving these next words special emphasis, "I strongly suggest that you talk to your mother."

CHAPTER 6

I AM NOTHING IF not a diligent student. I take my homework seriously.

I track my migraines, but it's hard to find a pattern. I can get a headache while dropping Nate off in his classroom, during lunch duty or my last-period class, picking Daniel up from Afterschool, getting the boys into bed at night. Or at four a.m., I might wake up from a dream in which my head is being crushed by boulders. I might find myself downing Excedrin before a date night with Stewart, trying to keep the pain at bay so I can maintain a compartment of myself for marital bliss and carefree sex. I might think about Matt, and the nausea will rise as light flashes behind my eyeballs. I'll be forced into bed and will cry under the covers, hoping I can purge my tears as well as my headache before the kids find me.

And my last surefire way to enter the migraine zone? Thinking about my other two assignments.

Why do I want an open marriage?

And do I really have to talk to my mother?

I ask Stewart to take the boys to the playground on a Saturday so I can call her. Earlier in the week, I sent an email asking if we could make time to talk. My mother and I speak on the phone regularly. So my request is designed to forewarn her: this won't be a typical chat.

Of course, she writes back. *How intriguing!*

I rack my brain for days, trying to think of where to begin. And I silently rehearse as she answers the phone, fumbling the receiver, reminding me again of her new physical reality.

"Hi, Mom!" I say, summoning my best cheerful voice.

"Hello, sweetie," she says, sounding like she's far away. "I'm sorry. Just give me one moment while I get the phone in the right spot."

It takes me back to phone calls with my grandmother in the months before she died. As often as not, the phone was upside down in her hand, and we'd have to shout at her to turn it around. At least my mother is aware of her issues.

"That's better!" Her voice is slower than it used to be but chipper as ever. "So what's going on? Your email got me so curious."

I take a deep breath, and before I lose my nerve, I spout the opening I've practiced: "Well, I'm seeing a therapist now, and he gave me homework to do. One of my assignments is to talk to you about something. But I'm not sure how to say it."

"I see!" she says. Sometimes I think my mother must be from central casting—she could have auditioned for the role of June Cleaver. "Well in that case, I suggest you just say it!"

While I'd guessed that my mother would respond like this, I'd never managed to script my next line. I take a deep breath and out tumbles an avalanche of unplanned words.

"Um, okay. So Stew wanted me to sleep with somebody else a few years ago like Dad told you that you should have an affair and so I did it his name is Matt and it went on for a while but now he doesn't want to talk to me anymore and I think Stewart and I are still fine but I'm worried that I might have ruined my marriage and I don't think I should ever do anything like this again except there were parts of it that were really nice and I miss Matt a lot but I don't know if I really miss him or if I just miss the way he made me feel and I still love Stewart but I don't think I can handle him being with other women and now I'm a mess and I have migraines all the time and I don't know what to do."

The moment I come up for air, I begin to sob. I'm not sure how much my mother has been able to decipher, but I can no longer speak. I cradle the phone between my left shoulder and ear and reach for the box of tissues by my bed.

"Oh, sweetie," my mother begins. "You've been holding this in for a long time. I'm so glad you're talking to me about it now."

"You are?" I snuffle. "I was afraid to tell you. The last time I brought up, you know, you and Jim, you seemed really . . . uncomfortable." I avoid calling it shame. Over a decade later, that conversation is still wrapped in the haze of postpartum exhaustion. But when I peel away the gauze that covers my own memory, I see my mother's stiff shoulders. I hear her halting words: *I was a virgin when we married. Your father thought an affair would give me confidence. It was a long time ago.*

"I suppose I was," she says. "And I'm still not eager to share intimate details about myself. But if *you* need to talk about it— well, that's different."

"Okay," I say. "I guess I don't really want to discuss details either. But I have a couple of questions. Just in general."

"All right," she says. "Ask away."

"Do you think sleeping with other people will ruin my marriage?"

"Definitely not," my mother says with such certainty that I laugh. She laughs, too. I'm reminded again of the sound of her laughter—like a ringing bell—when she used to talk to Jim on the phone. This is my real mother. Not the goody-two-shoes persona I tried to emulate throughout my childhood, but a whole person, one who defied the rules, is urging her daughter to do the same, and is laughing about it to boot.

"But how can you be so sure?" I say when we settle down.

"Because you and Stewart have the two magic ingredients," she says. "You talk to each other, and you love each other. If you keep doing those two things, opening yourself up to new experiences can only make your marriage richer and stronger."

"You make it sound so easy. Was it easy for you and Dad? Didn't you get jealous?" I ask, fishing for information. "I mean, I'm assuming he had your permission to sleep with other people, too."

"I'm not going to talk about your father's experience," my mother says, always the vault. Her words come out deliberately, with little pauses in between as she works to control the muscles of her mouth. "That's a conversation you'll need to have with him yourself." I cringe at the mere thought of asking my father about his sex life or sharing even a shred of information about my own. "I'll just say this: it was *not* easy. Not one little bit. We sometimes stayed up all night talking things through. But if I had to do it over again, I wouldn't change a thing."

A little lump of sadness rises in my throat as she says this.

"But, Mom," I say, "you had a real connection with Jim. And you're still friends with him. Maybe that's why you don't have any regrets. Matt and I barely ever saw each other. And I'm wondering now if it was all just—I don't know—superficial."

"Oh, sweetheart," says my mother. "Don't you worry. There will be more."

It doesn't hit me until I'm hanging up the phone: there must have been more for my mother as well.

That night, after the kids are in bed, Stewart sits me down on the couch and asks me about the conversation.

"How did it go?" he says, looking like he just scored backstage passes at a Van Halen concert. "What did you find out? Anything scandalous?"

"Not really," I say. "My mother always keeps it pretty vague."

He sighs and shakes his head in disappointment. "So what did you talk about?"

"We just talked about open marriage in general, although she never calls it that. I doubt she even knows the term." I pause, thinking of what else to say. I can't tell Stew I asked my mother whether she thought our marriage was in trouble. It would reveal my own fear. The irony is not wasted on me when I choose to focus on something else: "She did say you and I are good communicators. That's what's most important."

"Aw, that's sweet," says Stewart. "And I happen to agree." He squeezes my knee and kisses me. "I'm going to get some work done. Good night, my sexy Suitcase." Suitcase is his nickname for me. *Maleta* is one of the few words he remembers from high school Spanish, and to Stew, it sounds like *Molly*. My husband's mind is an interesting place.

"Good night, baby. I love you."

Later, I lie in our bed and think about my parents in theirs, during the years of my childhood. *We sometimes stayed up all night talking,* my mother had said. I remember overhearing at least some of these conversations. I could never make out the words, but the tone of their blended voices—my father's baritone and my mother's alto—was always a comfort to me. And now my mom believes that *I* have learned, through osmosis perhaps, the importance of communication in my own marriage.

But an unformed thought hovers at the edge of my mind. I'm starting to believe that this is the real source of my migraines—unspoken truths that I refuse to acknowledge, even to myself. The thought is starting to take shape now. It's about what my mother said to me, in the early days of her ataxia symptoms, as she began to slow down and stumble, to garble her words and drool.

Maybe it's all my repressed rage, she'd said.

How does that rage fit into the picture of marital harmony she's painted for me? A life in which she and my father gave each other freedom and talked through all their difficult feelings? Where did that rage come from?

And what does my mother's rage mean for me?

I BRING THESE QUESTIONS to my next session with Mitchell.

"What do *you* think is the source of your mother's rage?" he asks me.

And I'm back in 1979. My father comes home from a trip with his students. He leads an experiential education program for high school seniors. My mom is a teacher, too, but the "normal" kind, with classes to teach and papers to grade. The kind who is also a mother and has to pick up her kids and shop for groceries and make dinner and wash the dishes. My mother sighs heavily when my dad announces he's dropping off his laundry and leaving again the next day.

"That's the only way my mom ever expressed her anger," I tell Mitchell. "She sighed. I mean, how fucked up is that?"

"And how do you express *your* anger, Molly?" Mitchell asks.

Suddenly it clicks.

"I don't! That's why I get migraines!"

"Ahh," says Mitchell. "I think we're onto something. Did you track your headaches like I asked you to?"

"Yeah," I say. I've never been so excited to think about my headaches. I've taken notes on my phone. I open the document and start to read aloud. Nearly everything on my list—taking care of the kids, teaching, even sex with Stewart—has to do with a feeling of obligation. The only other item—thinking about Matt—relates to the disappearance of one thing in my life that *didn't* feel obligatory.

"I know men have obligations, too," I say, "but I'm pretty sure that being a mother feels different than being a dad. It's not just the duty to provide for your family. It's like, as a mother, you're supposed to give up your whole *self,* like you're not allowed to have a self at all."

"That's not an uncommon way for women to feel. And it sounds like your mother modeled this type of femininity for you—with one exception."

"Right! It's like sexual freedom was her only outlet," I say. "But she still blames her illness on *repressed rage.* So clearly that outlet wasn't enough."

"Molly," says Mitchell, leaning in with his elbows on his knees. "It seems you have an opportunity here. What can you learn from your mother's journey? Repressed emotion may have contributed to her illness. And repressed emotion seems very connected to illness in you as well—these debilitating migraines."

I meet his gaze and nod furiously, tears filling my eyes. It's such a relief to have someone spell out what the hell is going on with me.

"I'm going to give a name to the part of you that feels these obligations and represses anger—let's call her Straight-A Molly."

I laugh. "That definitely fits."

"And since Straight-A Molly loves homework, let's give her some. Our theme today is freedom. So I'd like you to fill out three lists."

He tears a fresh piece of paper from his notebook and writes at the top "REASSIGNING STRAIGHT-A MOLLY." Below the heading, he creates three columns. I love this assignment already. The block letters, the straight lines. This is my jam.

"The first column," Mitchell continues to narrate, "is 'FREE-DOM FROM.' . . . What does Straight-A Molly need to free herself from? Next is 'FREEDOM TO BE.' . . . And finally, 'FREEDOM TO DO.' " He finishes writing and gives the paper to me. It feels like he's handing me an actual piece of freedom.

"Great work today, Molly," Mitchell says. "I'll see you in two weeks."

I CARRY MY FREEDOMS in my pocket everywhere I go. By the end of the second week, the paper is the consistency of a used tissue, the writing almost illegible. I've crowded each column with freedoms I desire, and before I go back to Mitchell's office, I take stock, try to create some order from this formless chaos. I type my final list into my phone so I'll always have it with me.

FREEDOM FROM:
- pressure to be punctual
- self-imposed obligations (Never agree to be class parent again!)
- guilt
- pleasing others

FREEDOM TO BE:
- spontaneous
- imperfect
- my own priority
- honest with Stewart

FREEDOM TO DO:
- stupid shit
- things that are fun and just for me (guitar lessons?)
- a job that gives me more freedom than teaching

AT OUR NEXT SESSION, Mitchell praises my lists and encourages me to share them with Stewart. I've discovered that I like thinking of myself in the third person—as two people, in fact. Fuck Straight-A Molly. True Molly needs more freedom, more spontaneity, more imperfection, more, more, more!

After talking it over with Stew, I decide to quit teaching and take a job working as a curriculum writer and teacher trainer at the company my father founded when he retired from the classroom. It's a job that will include a bit of travel but is also part-time. Stewart vows to step up when I go out of town, and I imagine the freedom of going to the gym or Brooklyn Guitar School in the mornings, of grocery shopping on a weekday, of taking a plane by myself for "work trips."

We also decide to keep the marriage open. I'm determined to make open marriage work for me, to expand my sexual horizons and bring more spontaneity and adventure into my life. But despite my new focus on freedom, it's hard for an anxious leopard to change her sensible spots. I'm excited but also scared—scared of getting hurt, scared of losing Stewart. I tell Stew all of this. At the end of my monologue, I say:

"I don't think we should keep our old arrangement, though— that I'm supposed to tell you everything, but you don't tell me anything. Because if you don't tell me who you're with, I know I'm going to invent things. Like, I'll be scared that I know her, or that she's much younger than I am, or that you wish you were married to her instead of to me."

"Molly, that's not going to happen," Stew says. "But I have an idea. Let's set some new rules."

"Like, no ex-girlfriends?" Lena's divorce has been finalized, and she's dating someone new, someone who wants monogamy.

"Sure, I can do that."

Once I get started, my rules snowball. I don't write them down. Somehow saying them aloud is enough. I feel like I'm giving Stewart a script, but one that lives and breathes and can be changed as needed. *Here's how you need to behave so that I feel safe,* my rules are saying. But they also serve to highlight my every fear and insecurity:

Don't date an ex. Don't date anyone in the neighborhood. Don't date anyone too far away. Don't date someone you work with. No falling in love. Only go out on a date on a night when I also go out on a date. No going to anyone's house. No daytime dates. No sleeping over. No dating anyone you even might fall in love with. No playing chess or seeing movies with anyone else—those are our things. Don't date anyone too young. Don't show me pictures of her for a year. Tell me a little bit, but not too much. I'm serious: no falling in love. Only tell me the bad things. Don't text me right after a date because I'll be worried that you're still thinking about her. Never mind, do text me so I know you're thinking about me.

And remember: absolutely no falling in love.

A FEW WEEKS LATER, I'm out to dinner with my friend Edie, the mother of one of Daniel's classmates who I've long admired. She's stylish and sexy and so un-mom-like. Perhaps her key attribute is being single. This fact alone makes her one of the few people I can imagine telling about Stewart's and my arrangement.

I wait until we've ordered our second bottle of wine and then steer the conversation cautiously, focusing only on *her* experience.

"So what's dating like these days?" I ask.

"Oh my God," she says. "It's both amazing and awful. I just got on Tinder."

"What's that?"

"It's a dating app. Here, I'll show you."

Edie pulls out her Android and positions it so I can see.

"Here are all the single dudes within a five-mile radius. You swipe right if you like them, and swipe left if you don't." She starts showing me her options. Men of all shapes and colors scroll past. The one thing they apparently have in common is being under the age of thirty. "I'm addicted. This shit is like crack."

"Have you gone out with any of these guys?" I ask.

"I wouldn't exactly call it going *out*," she says, lifting her eyebrows significantly and making me laugh. "There's one guy who's been coming over to the house while the kids are at school. The sex is amazing, but he's so much younger than I am. Now he's totally in love with me. And I really don't want anything serious. It's a mess."

I can't decide if Edie is my hero or if she's waving a red flag. Maybe both. But she seems like the right person to ask for advice.

"So I have a question for you . . . ," I begin. I tell her about Matt and Lena, about my parents, about Stewart and me wanting to keep our marriage open in a way where nobody gets hurt. "Plus, I feel like I have to be discreet. I don't want the world to know."

This feels like a major stumbling block. The thought of other people learning about my shenanigans quite literally gives me hives. What would my next-door neighbor the pastor think if he knew I was a sexual infidel? Aside from Edie, would the upright moms of my sons' friends still let their kids sleep over at the house of a hussy? I'm even afraid of what the folks behind the counter of my pharmacy would think if they saw me buying condoms or—gasp!—*lube*.

"I get it," says Edie. "People can be so judgy." Then a light bulb goes off somewhere above her head. "Wait, do you listen to Howard Stern?"

"Uh, no," I say, refilling our wineglasses. My only association with Howard Stern is that he's a misogynistic asshole. But I'm trying to keep an open mind.

"He always talks about this dating website on his show," Edie continues. "It's called Ashley Madison. It's for people who are cheating. But, you know, sometimes guys aren't married, or they have a don't ask, don't tell policy with their wife, or something like that. You should check it out!"

The wine blends with Edie's encouragement to create what feels like genuine enthusiasm for this idea. Freedom from guilt, right? Freedom to be spontaneous! Freedom to do stupid shit! Plus, the chances of falling in love with an adulterer seem slim to none.

That night, drunk on a heady combination of wine and freedom, I go online and create an Ashley Madison profile. The site's tagline is *Life is short. Have an affair.* It's costly for men to join but free for women. Most of the clientele use fake names—Up-For-Anything, Scorpioman, Kinky4U—and include either below-the-neck pictures or doctored images. Their faces are covered in cartoonish tools of disguise—mustaches, sunglasses, and hats—provided by Ashley herself. I choose a photo Stew considers particularly sexy—I'm in a black dress and a Kentucky Derby hat, standing coquettishly on our front stoop—and then block out my eyes with a rectangle designed for this purpose. I name myself Mercedes Invierno, an alter ego constructed from my eighth-grade-Spanish-class handle and a spicy, roll-off-the-tongue translation of my surname. The twin sins of cultural appropriation and misrepresenting myself to men with Latina fetishes hardly seem important in the world of Ashley Madison.

Mercedes Invierno is a badass—Straight-A Molly's polar opposite. Within twenty-four hours of her debut on the online dating stage, Mercedes has gotten "likes" from over a hundred nameless, nearly faceless men, looking to *hook up* with a *partner in crime.*

And she eats up the attention like a warm plate of churros.

PART TWO

CHAPTER 7

IT'S THREE O'CLOCK ON a Wednesday somewhere along Amsterdam Avenue. I've arrived at one of the last seedy strongholds on the Upper West Side. A few lone daytime drinkers, wearing flannel and sadness, slump at the bar, where a tawny-haired woman in a too-small tank top refills their glasses. There is only one person seated at a table, toward the back where daylight can't reach. He's wearing a baseball cap and looks like one of the boys I used to see at parties in college. Good-looking but nondescript, the kind who was always with a skinny blond sorority girl and never glanced my way.

This is my date, Mike—although I doubt that's his real name. He watches me walk toward him and stands up tentatively.

"Mercedes?" he says, pronouncing it like the car.

"My real name is Molly," I say. God, I'm bad at this. "You must be Mike."

"Um, yeah, hi," he says, not correcting me. Definitely not his name. "I can't believe you're really you. I mean, you're just like your picture." He doesn't hide the fact that he's looking me up and down. But given the circumstances, why should he?

I laugh. "Is that usually not the case?"

"Oh God, you have no idea. Can I get you a drink?"

"I'll have whatever you're having," I say, nodding at the nearly empty beer in his hand.

"Cool." He heads to the bar. I sit down at the table and note with surprise how calm I feel. In control. I might have told Not-Really-Mike my real name, but Mercedes Invierno is the one who's here, the one who feels a stranger's eyes on her from twenty feet away and plays with her hair, crosses her legs, reapplies some lip gloss.

Not-Really-Mike comes back and sets down two glasses. He hesitates before he takes a seat beside me. But he won't make eye contact. He's nervous, and this adds to my feeling of power.

"So tell me about these women who aren't who they claim to be," I say as he takes a long swig.

"Oh God," he says again. "It's terrible. For men, at least. Half the 'women' on Ashley Madison are, like, Russian hackers or something. They just try to string you along and make up some crisis or another so you'll send them money. But if you suggest actually meeting, they put you off." He glances at me sideways to make sure I'm grasping the enormity of his hardship. "But that's not what I fell for."

I think about my AM inbox. Sorting through the dozens of men who write me every day has become something of a part-time job. No wonder I'm so popular. "Wow, I had no idea. So, what happened to you?"

"Well, I've only been on one other actual date," he says, gaining confidence as his tale lands as intended. "And her picture was super hot. It was taken recently, too, 'cause I could see a billboard from the latest James Bond movie in the background."

"Yeah?" I say in my most encouraging tone.

"But then when she showed up, she was, like, thirty years older than she was in the picture. Like the same person but thirty years *older*. It was so trippy. 'Cause how did she take that picture with the Bond billboard? It didn't look doctored or *anything*." Mike is gazing into the middle distance now, like he still can't fathom the *Twilight Zone* plot of his previous attempt at infidelity.

"That's super weird," I agree.

"And I didn't know what to say. I didn't want to be like, 'How'd you get so old so fast?' 'Cause that would be rude, you know?"

"Totally rude."

"So I was just like, 'You look kinda different from your picture,' and you know what she said to me?" He leans forward, exhaling eau de whiskey. I realize that, while I'm about to have my first drink, Mike has been at this bar for a while. I also notice his biceps rippling under his T-shirt, which seems to negate my first observation.

"What?"

"She says, 'Yeah, that picture I posted is of my daughter. But everyone says we look exactly alike!'" He shakes his head at the memory of it and takes another long sip of his drink. "How's that for some fucked-up shit?"

"That's pretty fucked up, all right."

"And by the way, before we keep talking about my shitty-ass life, I just have to say, you're gorgeous. Way hotter than that lady's daughter, even."

And there it is. The validation I crave.

A COUPLE HOURS LATER, Not-Really-Mike and I leave the bar and go for a stumbly walk in Central Park. The trees are awash in surreal yellows and reds; even the air is bright. People from another world—men in suits, women in pencil skirts—walk past us on their way home from work. I still have no idea what Not-Really-Mike does for a living that allows him to be out with me in the middle of the day, but I don't care. I glance at my phone to make sure the boys' school hasn't called. No voice mail, which means the sitter picked them up from Afterschool on time. I wonder if Stew ever checks his phone when he's on a date, if he stops to consider where the boys are at a given moment in time, if he feels the tug of responsibility taking him out of a hedonistic moment. But I already know the answer. He doesn't need to feel responsible because I've got it covered. I always have.

I grab Not-Really-Mike's hand and lead him off the paved path and onto the leaf-strewn grass. It's a classic rom-com scene—autumnal dusk in Central Park—in every way but one, and I feel like an alt-universe Meg Ryan. I stop at a huge elm tree, pull him toward me, let him pin my body against the ridged bark and guide his hand down the front of my jeans. I allow the anonymity of New York City to fall over me like a protective sheath, but even this brazen display doesn't feel reckless enough.

"Wait a sec," I say, or is that Mercedes Invierno's breathy voice I hear? I pull my phone from my back pocket. Besides clueing me in to the existence of Ashley Madison, Edie has also told me of another site where you can book a discounted hotel room for a few hours during the day. After a search for participating hotels on the Upper West Side—clearly the work of Straight-A Molly—I have a list of numbers in my phone. I call one now, give my credit card information on the spot, and suddenly, for the bargain-basement price of fifty-nine dollars, we have a room to go to. Not-Really-Mike stands back, watching me with almost as much disbelief as I watch myself.

At the hotel, I stop at the desk for the key. This involves handing over my driver's license, running my credit card for incidentals, initialing a document to show my understanding of the hotel's no-smoking policy. I'm sobering up too quickly and I fear Not-Really-Mike is, too. He stands apart from me, gazing around the lobby like he's looking for someone else. We claw at each other in the elevator, trying to rekindle our drunken passion, but once in the room, I realize I have to pee and rush wordlessly into the bathroom. I run the water in the sink to mask the sound of a potential fart and leave my jeans and shirt in a pile on the floor.

When I come out, Not-Really-Mike is lying on the bed. He is also stripped down to his underwear, and he tries to resurrect his erection with one hand, tries to pretend that whatever momentum we gained in the park hasn't been lost to reality. The lights are off, and the room is almost dark, the last hour of sunlight outlining the drawn window shades. In the dimness, I can look at him now, I can turn Not-Really-Mike into anyone I want. I climb onto the bed and straddle him, lean forward to kiss him while he fumbles with my bra clasp. I wonder if he has children, if his wife's breasts, like mine, are mottled with stretch marks, two semi-deflated balloons. I roll over onto my back so that I'm working with gravity, not against it. Even in the darkness, I feel exposed.

"Hang on," I say, the first words to leave my mouth since I spoke to the desk clerk. I reach for my bag and produce a box of condoms, further evidence that this plan isn't as spontaneous as I want Not-Really-Mike to believe. He dutifully opens the box as I stroke his penis, which is smaller than either Stewart's or Matt's. By the time he gets the condom on and manages to put himself inside me, he is already growing flaccid.

"I'm sorry," he mumbles. "It's been a while since I had to wear one of these. My wife is on the pill."

"Don't worry," I say. I let his cock flop out, peel off the condom in what I hope is a sexy, nonjudgmental way, and begin to lick the shaft like a melting ice pop. The room is poorly ventilated, and a few errant hairs plaster themselves uncomfortably to my lip. I prop myself up on one elbow so my sweaty chest won't stick to his legs and use the other hand to assist my mouth. I'm feeling confident now, more in my element. Blow jobs are something of a specialty of mine. When I went to college at age sixteen, I knew I wasn't ready to lose my virginity. My sister had gotten pregnant at nineteen, and intercourse scared me. But oral sex? That I could handle. I gave blow jobs to guys I met in my dorm, at fraternity parties, in Daytona Beach over spring break. I didn't savor the act, per se, but I relished the power I felt. Taking a penis in my mouth rather than my vagina gave me a sense of control.

But my endurance isn't what it used to be, and as my tired mouth continues to move up and down Not-Really-Mike's disappointing penis, as my drunken state starts to morph into the beginnings of a hangover, an uncomfortable feeling rises within me, a familiar and unwelcome sense of obligation. There is no way I can pretend I'm enjoying this. I'm only pumping my hand, taking him deeper into my mouth, so that he'll come sooner, so that this will be over.

Still, when Not-Really-Mike starts to moan, when he grabs my head in his hands and orgasms down my throat and I swallow it all, I do derive a kind of pleasure. I imagine that this is the first satisfying orgasm he's had in years, and I feel special. Afterward, I massage his naked, bristly back, and we engage in a parody of pillow talk.

"That was a lot of fun," he says.

"Yeah, it was," I lie.

"You were amazing," he says.

"Thanks," I say.

"I'd better get going if I'm going to catch my train," he says.

"Oh, where do you live?" I ask.

"Westchester," he answers vaguely.

"Well, thanks for coming into the city to meet me," I say.

"No problem at all," he says.

When he leaves, I look at the time on my phone. It's 7:23 p.m.—Daniel's time of birth. I quickly calculate Daniel's exact age in order to distract myself from the sadness that creeps into the room, threatening to envelop me as I lie naked on the bed. Daniel is twelve years, seven months, and fifteen days old. This is how long I've been a mother.

I think about Rachel Cusk's memoir about motherhood, *A Life's Work,* which a friend gave me after Nate was born. In the introduction, Cusk writes about childbirth dividing mothers from the rest of the world, dividing women even from themselves. The line I remember verbatim is this: "When she is with them she is not herself; when she is without them she is not herself; and so it is as difficult to leave your children as it is to stay with them." I feel this to be profoundly true. It seems impossible that the person who just fucked a stranger is the same person who Daniel and Nate call *Mom.* I don't even remember how to code-switch. I don't know how to return to a state of motherhood fast enough to relieve the babysitter and put my children to bed. So I stay motionless on the crumpled bedspread, which Not-Really-Mike and I never bothered to remove, and watch the lights of passing cars animate the blank wall. At nine thirty, it feels safe to leave—the kids should be asleep by now—and so I do.

"I THINK I NEED to date more than one person," I say to Mitchell after relaying the story of Not-Really-Mike. Now that over a week has passed, it feels like just that: a story. I'm sitting cross-legged on the couch, a Starbucks pumpkin latte in my hand, speaking casually, as if Mitchell has fallen behind in his reading for book club and I'm catching him up on the pages he missed.

"And why is that?" he asks.

I've prepared my answer to this question.

"I don't want to get too hung up on any one guy." Not-Really-Mike waited two full days to text a lukewarm invitation to repeat my first performance: *Can't stop thinking about your mouth, wanna hook up again?* I didn't even like him. I could admit that much to myself. But I still felt disappointed by his delayed response, by the reference to nothing more than my ability to give head. "I feel like if I date a few guys at a time, then it'll be easier to stay emotionally detached. That's what Stew does. He's dating, like, four different women right now."

Stew continues to be careful not to share details, but he does tell me who he's seeing and when. This information creates a strange mix of comfort and jealousy. On the one hand, if Stew is dating lots of women, he's unlikely to fall in love with any one of them. But on the other hand, I'm jealous of how easy it all seems for him.

"Okay," says Mitchell, taking his signature pause. I've discovered that he sometimes scrunches up his eyes at these moments, usually when he's trying to figure out the best way to say something I don't want to hear. His eyes are scrunched now. His thumb and index finger rest on his forehead to boot, emphasizing this look of concentration. "You've just told me that you're striving for 'emotional detachment' in your relationships with men. However, when you described your date with Mike, it sounded to me like detachment was part of what left you feeling so unfulfilled." He opens his eyes and looks at me. "Do you see the dilemma here?"

"Yeah." I sigh. "I guess so. Maybe what I really want is for men to feel attached to *me,* but for me to feel detached from *them.*"

"Ahh," says Mitchell, taking more notes. "Do you know what that says to me?"

"No," I answer honestly. But I can't wait to find out. Even when Mitchell delivers a difficult truth, I'm grateful for his ability to make sense of my contradictory parts.

"It says that you're still trying to please others in order to get validation for yourself. Do you see what I mean?"

"Not exactly," I say.

"Well, your date with Mike is a good example. You wanted him to desire *you,* and you wanted to please *him* sexually. That was more important to you than desiring *him* or deriving any real pleasure for yourself."

"Yeah, I guess that's true."

"And I'm not suggesting it's a bad idea for you to date more broadly," he continues. "However, I do think it's important to figure out what brings *you* pleasure. Maybe having multiple partners will be part of that. But as you've told me before, what works for Stewart won't necessarily work for you. You need to pay close attention to *yourself* and to what you are receiving or gaining from each relationship."

THAT NIGHT, I SPEND hours reading through my messages on Ashley Madison, of which there are hundreds. I'd gone out with Not-Really-Mike because he was good-looking and younger, two qualities that were supposed to make me feel better about my fortysomething self. But I see Mitchell's point. I need to raise my standards, to find men who have something to offer *me.* I end up making dates with two different men for the coming week.

First, I meet Leo, who isn't even married. His girlfriend of five years lives in Philadelphia, and he tells me they have an agreement: what they do on their separate turf is their own business. Leo is funny, a comedy writer who has worked on shows I like. He's a minor celebrity, with a page on IMDb and everything, assuring me of the truth of his identity. He invites me to a bar near his place in Hell's Kitchen.

I don't drink anymore, he writes, *but I don't mind watching you sip a cocktail or two.* This is the last time I see Leo anywhere other than his apartment.

Leo is older than I am, older than Stewart even, and his experience shows. He's a creative lover. One day I get a text asking me, *What is the sexiest song you can think of?*

Kiss, I write. And then, unnecessarily, *by Prince.*

The next time I go to Leo's, he meets me at the door with a pair of headphones and a bandanna. He ties the bandanna around my head, blindfolding me, then places the headphones over my ears. I hear the vibrations of the opening guitar riff, and by the time Prince has instructed me to leave it all up to him, Leo has slid my panties down to my ankles and is on his knees under my miniskirt.

After that, I never make it into Leo's bedroom fully clothed. The moment I come through the door, his hands are on me and he's kissing me deeply, unbuttoning my jeans or unzipping my dress.

He is deft with one-handed bra removal, with maneuvering me onto his bed while at least three fingers move inside me.

The first time Leo fists me, I have no idea what's happening. I feel a physical fullness unlike anything I've ever experienced. Afterward, I ask him to show me what he did, and I gasp as he points to a spot below his wrist.

"All of that was inside me?!"

"Yup," he says, enjoying my look of alarm.

"I didn't know that was possible!"

"Not everybody likes it as much as you do," he adds, stroking my thigh. "You're clearly into G-spot stimulation."

THEN THERE IS LAURENT. He's half French and half Argentine, a combination that sets him apart from the riffraff in my Ashley Madison inbox. If pleasure is my goal, how can I go wrong with that sexual pedigree? Unlike Leo, Laurent is in fact married and has two small children. But he assures me that he and his wife have a don't ask, don't tell agreement.

"She eez from Brazil," he tells me. "She has . . . how do you say . . . an understanding of Latin men."

On our first date, Laurent follows me into the women's bathroom and fingers me as I sit on the sink. On our second date, he follows me again and I let him fuck me. On our third, I meet him on a corner in Chelsea and he says he has a surprise: tickets to a show.

"Really?" I say, perking up in a way that makes me admit something to myself: I've been craving real dates. From our credit card bills, I know that Stewart always takes women out to dinner before heading to a hotel. But I'm not Stewart, I tell myself. For me, dinner and detachment don't mix, right? "Like a Broadway show?"

He laughs. "Not quiiite. But you like Shakespeare, no?"

My heart jumps a bit higher. He remembers something I said on a previous "date." In the awkward moments after copulating in the bathroom, I made a joke about ticking items off my bucket list—*Next up, prison sex!*—then jabbered about an amazing production of *Julius Caesar* I'd seen, set in a women's penitentiary. I didn't think Laurent was even listening. On the contrary, he noted one of my passions, bought tickets, and made thoughtful plans for our evening.

Laurent takes my hand and walks purposefully. When he turns to steer me through the doors of a stately hotel, I take my hand away.

"Wait, what's going on?" I demand.

He laughs again. "You have heard of *Sleep No More,* no?"

"No," I admit. "What's that?"

"Eet eez a show. Based on *Macbeth.* You weel love it."

Laurent holds the door open, and I walk through the dimmed lobby, where two women in black masks and red gowns gesture toward the bar. Laurent gets wine for us while I look at the art deco chandeliers and brass railings and try to formulate a question. When he returns, all I can think to say is "Have you done this before?"

Laurent laughs again and holds a finger to his lips. It's then that I realize everyone is speaking in whispers. I drink my wine and watch the other patrons. No one else looks nearly as confused as I feel. The women in the red gowns beckon to us, and, silently, the small group convened at the bar follows them. We are brought to an old-fashioned elevator, and the women hand each of us a full-face white mask and glide wordlessly away. I pull mine on as an attendant ushers us inside, then closes the accordion-style gate. Looking at the identically masked faces that surround me, I feel less like I've arrived at a production of *Macbeth* and more like I've joined the cast of *Eyes Wide Shut*. There is something charged in the air. Something erotic. And dangerous.

As we start to ascend, the elevator attendant says in a throaty, theatrical voice: "Welcome to *Sleep No More*. Here, you must follow three rules: No talking, no cell phones, and no taking off your mask." The elevator abruptly stops and the doors open. "And remember," the attendant adds, "fortune favors the bold!"

Laurent takes my hand. He leads me through various spaces where actors pantomime scenes from the play, but out of sequence. I used to teach *Macbeth,* and I'm geeking out on the abstraction of it, trying to decipher the prophecies of the witches, the killing of Macduff's wife and son, but Laurent won't let me linger. He pulls me from one room to the next, down staircases, and finally toward a group of white-masked spectators gathered around a blood-spattered bathtub where a naked woman is washing herself. This is an easy one: Lady Macbeth after the killing of Duncan. I'm watching, mesmerized, when Laurent places my hand on his crotch and whispers in my ear, "Follow me."

He moves toward a dark corner where a red velvet curtain has been secured. He glances around before diving behind it, pulling me with him. The curtain weighs heavily against me. I feel like a corpse wrapped in a rug, a sensation worsened by the mask I wear. I take it off, but Laurent leaves his on, a specter floating before my straining eyes.

I hear his labored breath echoing behind the mask and glance at his hand, which is now down his pants, pumping away at his erection. With his other hand, Laurent pushes on my shoulder. I fall to my knees and Laurent puts his cock in my mouth. We are so close to the other audience members that I can hear their whispers, see their shoes. Within moments, Laurent is coming in my mouth. An instant later, he zips up and steps out from behind the curtain, leaving me there on my knees.

Never mind, I tell myself. I'm having adventures. I am *living*.

ONE DAY, LEO SENDS me a text: *Maybe you should get yourself a butt plug and bring it along next time. I have a feeling you'll enjoy it.* There's a sex shop in Park Slope called Babeland. I've always thought it looked out of place, flanked as it is by a children's bookstore and a vegan café. The idea of someone seeing me go inside is too horrifying to contemplate. But for reasons I can't explain, the idea of ordering a sex toy online is equally mortifying. I decide instead to take a field trip to the original Babeland on the Lower East Side, where mothers pushing strollers are as rare as—well, as mothers buying butt plugs.

I wander over to the anal-toy table and gasp at the length and girth of some of the items on display. There are anal beads that heat up, dildos that come with remote controls, plugs that attach to fuzzy bunny-rabbit tails. A tatted employee with a double nose ring helps me select a "starter butt plug"—it's purple, made of silicone, and frankly adorable. Even if the name of the store didn't give it away, it would be obvious this place is geared toward women.

"I recommend you also purchase some high-quality lube," the saleswoman adds, so I do. I'm glad I've brought my backpack, and I cram the bright pink Babeland shopping bag inside it as soon as I leave the store.

At home that night, after the kids are asleep, I decide to experiment with my new little toy. Lying on my bed with a bottle of lube at my side, I lift my tush onto a pillow and try to relax. I feel like I did the first time I inserted a tampon. My mother never discussed such things with me, so it wasn't until my freshman year of college that I gave it a try. I came back from our shared bathroom and told my roommate, a no-nonsense sophomore from Flint, Michigan, that the tampon wouldn't fit. Patiently, she drew a diagram of the three holes I possessed. I was embarrassed to admit I'd only been aware of two.

"The top one is for pee. It's right under your clitoris. The middle one is where you have sex—that's where the tampon goes. The bottom one is for poop." She handed the paper to me. "Don't come back until you've figured it out."

I did figure it out, and I'm determined to figure this out, too. The woman at Babeland recommended inserting a lubed finger into my own asshole first—then, when I relaxed around it, doing a switcheroo with the butt plug.

"Just wear it around the house at first—ten or fifteen minutes at a time," she said, "until you build up your endurance. But eventually, you should be able to wear it all day if you like. Some people even sleep with them."

The idea of wearing a butt plug for twenty-four hours is about as appealing as getting my appendix pierced. But knowing that some people treat their plugs like a comfy pair of slippers has piqued my curiosity. And after a few attempts, it's in.

It's a strange sensation, to be sure—not bad, and maybe even good.

Stewart is downstairs working in his studio, and I send him a text: *Do you know what I'm wearing?*

I'm guessing it's not a muumuu, he answers.

Come upstairs and see, I tease.

Let me just lay down this track. I'll be right there.

By the time Stew makes it to the bedroom, I'm starting to chafe. But I want credit for my daring, so I bend over and show him my little purple protrusion.

"What the hell is that?" he asks.

"It's my new sex toy!" I say.

He looks at me strangely. "I didn't know you were into that."

"Well, I'm still not sure if I am. It was Leo's idea, but I wanted to try it out at home first."

"I thought Laurent was the kinky one."

"They're both kind of kinky, I guess," I say, growing annoyed. "But what do *you* think?"

"I don't know," says Stewart, then pauses. "Is this supposed to be some kind of invitation?"

"That's what I was thinking when I texted you, but now it's starting to hurt," I say. When I see the confusion on his face, inarticulate anger rises within me. "Why did you take so long to come upstairs?" I shout.

"Why are you angry at me?" he shouts back. "You bought a sex toy to use with your boyfriend, and you're yelling at me because I didn't come up fast enough to test-drive it?"

The words come out before I have a chance to think about them.

"I'll bet you took your time because you're so tired from having sex with a million other women that you don't want to have sex with me!"

"A million women?" says Stewart, sitting down on the bed next to me and sighing. "I'm glad you think I'm such a Casanova, Molly, but that's a slight exaggeration, don't you think?"

"It all just seems so easy for you," I blurt, finally saying what I've been thinking for months. Mercedes Invierno wants to pretend that sex with multiple men is a dream come true. And Straight-A Molly is too competitive to admit that Stewart is winning the Open Marriage Games. I lean against Stew, wearing my best pout.

Stew puts an arm around me. "You know why that is, right?"

I look at him sideways, suspicious of what's coming next. "Why?"

"Because I date *women,*" he says. "And you date *men*. And as we both know, *men suck.*"

"True," I say. I feel some of the tension leave my body. It's a relief to fall into arms that know exactly how I like to be held.

"And for the record," he says, pulling me in, "I *do* want to have sex with you. You just took me by surprise."

"I've been taking *myself* by surprise," I mumble into his chest. "What the hell is going on with me?"

"Oh, baby, don't worry. I'm here to help you figure it out. But first, there's something you have to learn all by yourself."

I snuggle in closer. "And what's that?" I like the idea that Stew knows me so deeply. What will he say? That I need to learn to trust my voice? To set clearer boundaries? To put my self-respect above my need to please?

He looks down at me, and his deadpan expression starts to break. "You need to learn how to take out a butt plug," he says, and bursts into laughter.

CHAPTER 8

I TELL MITCHELL ABOUT Laurent, about Leo, about my argument with Stew. I leave in the part about buying a butt plug—it
feels like a clinical purchase, yet to be put to real sexual use—but
I leave out the settings of my trysts with Laurent, the fisting with
Leo. Something stops me from getting graphic with Mitchell.

"So, Molly," Mitchell begins when I've finished my summary.
"I think we have two different issues going on here."

"Only two?"

Mitchell laughs. "We'll start with two. For one, it sounds like
you're feeling a disconnect between your sexual self and the rest of
you. And second, it seems you're afraid that Stewart's relationships
will interfere with your marriage, particularly when it comes to
sex."

Damn he's good.

"I wonder, though," Mitchell continues, "if it's possible for
you and Stewart to use your sexual exploration outside marriage
to build a stronger bond with each other. I think your impulse to
invite Stew to experiment with a sex toy with you was a healthy
one. It shows you're willing to talk openly with him about new
sexual experiences you're having and your desire to integrate those
experiences into your marriage."

"I don't know if I'm ready to hear about Stewart's sexual exploration, though," I admit. "I don't want him lying to me, but I also

don't want to know any details about women he's dating. Or what he's doing with them."

"Tell him that. But it sounds like Stewart is open to hearing about *your* self-discovery. So maybe you should just start there."

"Okay," I say. "It's weird, though. Stew and I have always been able to talk about sex, or at least our sex with each other. I feel kind of embarrassed talking about sex that's not with him, especially some of the kinky stuff I'm trying."

"One person's kink is another's vanilla," says Mitchell. "From what you've told me about Stewart, it seems unlikely that you'll shock him."

I laugh. "True."

"But your embarrassment around talking with Stewart about sex brings me to the disconnect I mentioned earlier. Aside from your sexuality, you're not sharing much of yourself with either Laurent or Leo. I think it would be a great exercise for you to disclose more of who you are with them. You need to narrow the gap between Mercedes and Molly."

LAURENT CAN'T EVEN PRONOUNCE my name. He rhymes it with *holy*. Meanwhile, my Midwestern mouth flops open with a strangled gurgle on the final consonant of his name. Mostly we avoid calling each other anything at all. So I decide that Leo is a better candidate for sharing my true self.

Over the next weeks, instead of sexting with him like I usually do, I send Leo recordings of me singing and playing guitar. I invite him to one of my "gigs," which is just an open mic at a hole-in-the-wall Brooklyn bar. He tells me he'd love to come, but a few hours beforehand, I receive a text: *Tonight's a bust for me, but break a leg!* He suggests I learn a Joan Armatrading song that he thinks will suit my voice, and I spend hours working on it, eager to play it for him in person. The moment never arrives, but still, I feel like our connection has moved beyond sex. Leo offers me postcoital San Pellegrinos, which we drink standing naked in the small kitchen of his apartment, and the week after Christmas, he hands me a jar of the preserved lemons he'd given to all his friends as holiday gifts.

"They're great stuffed into a roast chicken," he tells me.

This means something to me. I am a person Leo can envision somewhere other than his bed, a person with such a full life that I might need an easy way to perk up chicken for a spur-of-the-moment dinner party.

On a languid Sunday afternoon in February, while Stewart takes Daniel and Nate to the movies, I'm lying in Leo's bed. The radiator of his prewar building blasts hot air, so we crack open the window. Delicious sensations of heat and cool creep over my sated body as Leo gazes at me from a propped elbow.

"So, MJ," he says, "I have a question for you." At some point, Leo and I started a game of guessing each other's middle names with only the first letter as a clue. I landed on Richard almost immediately. But after a couple of genuine tries—*Jennifer? Jocelyn?*—his guesses became more outrageous. *Jabba the Hutt? J.Lo?* Now he seems content to call me by my initials. I enjoy being MJ—like Spider-Man's girlfriend—which lies somewhere between the reality of Molly Jean and the fantasy of Mercedes Invierno.

"No, it's not Jambalaya," I say.

He laughs. "Good to know, but this is a real question. Where does your husband think you are right now?"

I answer reflexively—but I'm surprised that my reflex is to tell the truth. I guess MJ is closer to Molly than I thought.

"He knows I'm here. With you. We have an open marriage." Leo's eyes widen in surprise, and I hurry to add, "Sorry I never said anything. I was afraid it might bother you."

"No way," he says, moving his head somewhere between a

nod of affirmation and a shake of disbelief. "That's really fucking evolved. Sexy, too."

"Yeah?"

"Totally," he says. "And here I was, thinking I was corrupting you. But you've got it all worked out."

"I wouldn't go that far," I say. "I'm still getting used to it. In fact, you're one of the only people I've told."

"Well, I'm honored," he says. "I've thought about being more open with Claire about . . . everything. I'm sure she knows. But I guess I like the thrill of secrecy, you know?"

IN TERMS OF THEIR attraction to the illicit, I wonder if Leo and Laurent are more alike than I realized.

One day, I'm at Nate's school, where, in an attempt to tick a box on the Good Mother Checklist, I've joined a PTA committee. After our meeting ends, I head outside and reach for my phone to read my email. I see a message labeled URGENT: BREACH OF CONTRACT and hurry to open it.

> Dear Breather Client:
>   We regret to inform you that you have violated the Terms of Service regarding the prohibition of sexual activity in one of our Breather Spaces. The Breather Community is built around mutual trust and respect. Members who fail to follow our community norms are thus banned in perpetuity from further use of our Spaces. Furthermore, the credit card on file will be charged an additional $200.

I feel a sagging humiliation as I glance around to see if any of the "normal" mothers have noticed the pervert in their midst. I skitter into a shadowy corner of some nearby scaffolding and type out a text to Laurent.

I've just been banned from Breather! For life! And I'm being charged $200! WTF??

I watch as three dots appear underneath my message.

This is crazy, he replies. *Thank God we have used your credit card!*

I study his words and shake my head. Is he kidding? The fact that we find humor in very different things is just one issue that makes me wonder why I'm still dating Laurent. But whether he's joking or not, I'm waiting for a gesture from him, an offer to at least cover half of this unexpected expense. The whole idea of a Breather room had been Laurent's idea after all. True, he would have happily continued having sex in bar bathrooms, but when I complained that it was getting old, he suggested we do the deed in a Breather room—one of the office spaces sprinkled throughout the city where one can work, hold a meeting, or, as the website says, *simply recharge.* Laurent assured me that a pay-by-the-hour structure was coded permission to recharge in whatever way we saw fit. He asked me to book the room so his wife wouldn't see it on their credit card bill.

"Zhe knows, but zhe dooz not want to know, you see?"

So I created a Breather account, added a credit card, and booked the room.

But as it turns out, Breather rooms are not intended for lascivious use. I'm still wondering how they know about my breach, my violation, my flagrant disrespect for *community norms.* Was there a video camera hidden alongside the sterile artwork on the walls, under the wood-veneer desktop, on the leather swivel office chair? Or were there neighbors who heard our sex sounds and complained? I also wonder if the fee is a punishment or if it's the cost of the deep cleaning required to wash away the stain of sin. In truth, I don't want to know more than I already do—I'm banned, my card is being charged an extra two hundred dollars, and Laurent is expressing nothing but relief.

"So I got a pretty crazy email today," I say to Stewart as we get ready for bed.

"Did someone find your butt plug?" He's been teasing me ever since I got home from a date with Leo and discovered that I'd left the bag with my plug and lube on the subway.

"Haha." I punch him lightly on the shoulder. I tell Stew about the Breather fine, about being banned, and he laughs.

"This is way better than the Tale of the Lost Butt Plug. Pun intended."

I roll my eyes.

"Why don't you guys just get a hotel? He can afford it."

I've told Stewart that Laurent is a "finance guy," but I've skipped over some other relevant information. Although he's six years my junior, Laurent is already on his third marriage and spends a huge amount of money each month on alimony. Regardless, I bristle at what sounds to me like a sexist assumption about who should be paying for dates. I know Stew pays for every hotel room, every dinner—with the occasional exception when a woman insists. I suspect he harbors the notion that this is the way it should be, though he'd never say it outright.

"I think Laurent likes it to feel a little taboo," I answer.

This isn't the only thing he likes that's taboo. As Mitchell suggested, I tell Stewart everything, just as he's always wanted, in a kind of fever pitch. Things like: "Sometimes Laurent slaps my face and then licks my cheek. It actually feels good!" Stew looks at me through squinted eyes, trying to make sense of the unrecognizable person before him.

Once, Stewart and I are having sex, and I ask him to turn me onto my belly so he can enter me from behind, the way Laurent does.

"Flip me!" I moan.

Confused, but trying to go with the flow, Stewart smacks my face. Not hard, but enough to shock me into tears.

"Why did you do that?" I sob.

"You told me to hit you!" he objects. "I thought you liked that now!"

"I said 'Flip me,' not 'Hit me!'" I shout at him. "And anyway, I only like it when Laurent does it."

I'M BENT OVER MY desk, standing on tiptoe to improve Laurent's angle and trying not to hit my head on the computer monitor, when I hear a *ding,* the opening of elevator doors. Laurent is busy making his own sounds, grunting behind me.

"Shh," I whisper. "I think someone's coming."

"Eet is ukay," says Laurent, not missing a stroke. "Joost relax."

Cubicle sex is decidedly *not* relaxing. Even so, I've brought Laurent to my shared Greendesk workspace in Dumbo, a cheaper by-the-month version of Breather, where care for the environment is expressed by never turning on the air-conditioning or heat. Because of the late hour, as well as the unseasonably cold weather, I assumed my floor would be empty of all witnesses and my plexiglass-enclosed cubicle would provide an adequate setting for a quickie.

But now I'm hearing voices. And they're headed toward us, entering the cubicle two doors down. Laurent doesn't stop. And I don't ask him to.

"Ouiiiii," he moans.

I keep my head positioned so the monitor hides most of my face. But in my mind's eye, I picture my work neighbors, two tall guys and a nerdy woman with glasses, who occupy the large corner office. I don't know their names, but I sometimes make small talk with the woman at the copier. Although their voices are muted, the conversation flows without interruption. The lights above my desk are off—maybe we can evade detection.

As Laurent's thrusts gain momentum, I push my feet into the floor and my ass into his pelvis as hard as I can. My own pleasure is no longer the objective. I need him to come quickly so I can plan our escape. Just as I hear Laurent reach his peak—"Oooohhhh!"— I hear something else that makes my legs turn liquid. Silence. I bury my face in my forearms.

Laurent flops forward and breathes heavily onto my back. But the normal rhythm of conversation at the end of the hall has stopped. And then: whispers.

"Moly, that wuz fantastique," pants Laurent.

"Shhhhhh . . . ," I say again, weakly. "I think they heard us."

Laurent laughs without adjusting his volume. "Yoo Americainz are too serious! What eez de problem wiz a leetle luv-makeeng?"

I hear the elevator doors again and wait a beat before deciding it's safe to stand.

"Well, at least give me your condom so I can throw it away in the bathroom," I say, pulling up my jeans and turning around. "I don't want the cleaning staff to see it."

Laurent looks at me with a sheepish smile. "Oops," he says, raising his hand to his mouth with a faux gasp. "It zeems I have forgot zee condom!"

Pain is gathering around the crown of my head. This isn't the first time he's fucked me from behind without protection. The last time, he claimed his condom had fallen off. And now he's not even attempting to lie. But I should have known, shouldn't I? I should have been able to feel the difference. I stare at him, trying to decide which one of us is more to blame.

"Eet is okay, Moly," he says. "I em very cleen, yes? And you are on the pill, no?"

"That's not the point," I say. "Whatever. Let me at least go pee so I don't end up with another UTI."

I haven't told Stew about the no-condom incident, rationalizing that we both get tested for STDs regularly. But it's hard to hide a urinary tract infection from him. In the six months I've been dating Laurent, I've already had three. After the last one, Stew let out a resentful sigh. "This guy is breaking all my toys," he complained. Still, that's as far as he's gone in terms of criticism.

Laurent reaches for my hand as I move to open the cubicle door. The doors are pointless, really, since the so-called walls separating one compartment from the next don't even touch the ceiling.

"You go make a pee but I must leave. I em quite late."

I sigh. It's been weeks since we walked out of a building together. Laurent pulls me toward him and grabs my face with his other hand.

"*Bonne nuit, ma chérie,*" he says, kissing me. He releases my face with dramatic flair and grabs his jacket. "I weel call."

Without bothering to button my jeans, I stumble down the hall to the ladies' room. As I pee, I contemplate the roll of industrial toilet paper under the fluorescent bathroom lights. This is supposed to be about my fun, my pleasure, my freedom. How have I arrived at this point? I'm honestly not sure.

Shame will do that, smear the details until they become tolerable.

CHAPTER 9

SITTING ON THE PLANE, on my way to lead a teacher training somewhere outside Houston, I try to be subtle as I scratch my crotch.

A couple of weeks ago, Laurent asked me a rather pointed question: "Have you ever considered waxing?"

The French accent made it worse.

I was indignant. Who did he think he was, telling me what to do with my body? What kind of sicko would want me to look like a prepubescent girl? But my outrage was overshadowed by self-doubt.

I remembered hanging out in a dorm room during my freshman year of college with a group of newly minted men and women. It was one of those conversations that made you realize you weren't in high school anymore, and we moved from one revelation to another at titillating speed. My friend Rahul, who'd grown up without sisters in a conservative Indian family, had just had his mind blown—*A period can last for a week?!*—and a new question was posed: *If you could change one thing about yourself physically, what would it be?* I had my answer ready, and foolishly went first.

"I wouldn't have so much body hair," I said.

There was a shocked pause, followed by a burst of laughter. I don't remember what anyone else's answer was. Probably *I would have longer toes* or *I wouldn't be so skinny.*

Laurent had named the physical trait I hated most about myself, but I refused to give him the satisfaction of admitting it. Still, I decided to poll Stewart. I hoped his answer would provide some solace.

"So, do any of the women you've dated . . . wax . . . you know . . . their pussies?"

"Whoa!" he said. "Where did that come from?"

"Just answer the question."

"I guess the majority do."

"What?!" This was not the answer I'd hoped for.

"But not all. And not everyone gets a full Brazilian," he said hastily. "Plus, I really don't care one way or the other."

"Laurent cares," I said, dejected. "He basically asked me to get waxed. I thought he was some sort of perv, but I guess I'm the weird one."

"Baby, you're not weird. I *like* your bush," said Stew, giving me a come-hither look. Stewart can get turned on by *any*thing.

"It's not just my bush," I complained. "I've got so much hair on my upper thighs, and when I shave, it gets all red and bumpy. Maybe he's right. Maybe I should get rid of it."

"Do whatever you want, my little Hobbit," Stew said, kissing me on the head. "I'll think you're sexy either way."

I decided to at least check out my options and booked a consultation at V&N Laser Skin Care. Lasering seemed like a quicker fix than waxing—at least I wouldn't have to subject myself to torture every few weeks. But my hopes were quickly dashed. Either Valeria or Natalia, the practically identical Russian ladies who owned the operation, took one look at my pubes and clucked with disapproval. Bow-legged and mired in self-pity, I left the salon with nineteen sessions remaining from the twenty-pack I'd purchased. Pruning my particular landscape would apparently be a time-consuming, expensive, and painful enterprise.

But nobody warned me about the itching. I've spent the entire flight with a sweatshirt over my lap to hide my scratching fingers. And now, as the plane lowers toward the flat expanse of Houston, I work on a strategy to grab my suitcase from the overhead bin and bolt to the front of the plane. I need to get to the ladies' room so I can scratch freely and apply some witch hazel.

As we taxi to the gate, I reach for my phone to distract myself. I take it out of airplane mode and watch as a flurry of texts descends from cyberspace. They're all from Daniel.

And now, here I am, standing against the plaster wall of the terminal, squeezing my carry-on between my legs in an effort to scratch my labia against each other, and hearing the croak of Daniel's thirteen-year-old voice on the other end of the line.

"So—are you and Dad in an open marriage?"

The hand holding the phone shakes as I work to steady my voice.

"I want you to know something, Daniel. Dad and I are very happy together, and we're always honest with each other. He tells me everything, and I tell him everything."

Silence.

"Wait. You do it, too?"

"Well, it wouldn't be fair if it were just Dad," I splutter.

"Yeah, I was thinking that," replies my burgeoning feminist, "but I have a question."

"Shoot." I brace for whatever comes next.

"*When?* I mean, I get that Dad has time for it, but when do *you* do it?"

Daniel's question brings me relief on two levels. One, he's using the beautifully vague word *it*. *It* can mean anything. *It* can mean going out with other men in a purely social or intellectual way. *It* can mean that I'm out in the world, having deep conversations about poetry and politics, not fucking adulterers in bar bathrooms.

Two, I've worried that I'm not spending enough time at home, enough time with my children. And here is the affirmation that, in Daniel's mind at least, I'm around so often he can't fathom my managing to be anywhere else.

Still, I sidestep the question. In other words, I lie.

"I don't do it very often." I hope my tone is both breezy and convincing. But it seems like now would be a good time to redirect the conversation, so I ask Daniel to do something for me. "Could you please put away Dad's laptop? I don't want Nate to see it."

"Way ahead of you, Mom." The idea of his younger brother finding out about *it* is almost as abhorrent to Daniel as it is to me. While most kids—Daniel included—would rather avoid talking with their parents about sex, or would at least keep those talks as short and nebulous as possible, ten-year-old Nate is quite the opposite. He sees the world through a sexual lens and shares his observations with whomever is close at hand.

When Nate was only three, I picked him up from his preschool classroom. His teacher asked to speak with me for a moment outside.

"I took Nate and another student to the bathroom today," she said, barely containing her mirth. "And do you know what he said to her?"

I decided not to guess.

"He said, 'Your butt looks good!'" She broke into peals of laughter. I was relieved that Nate's statement was met with amusement rather than alarm.

When he was seven, I checked out some bedtime books at the library. One of them was titled *King & King*. It was about a prince who didn't want to marry a princess; he wanted to marry another prince instead. As the story progressed, Nate got increasingly wound up, giggling and squirming and being all kinds of silly. Fearing that I was raising a homophobic child, I reprimanded him.

"Nate," I said. "How would you like it if you wanted to marry a princess, and somebody forced you to marry a prince?"

His eyes twinkled. "I'd say, bring on the men!"

To Nate, sex was sex was sex. And it was all cause for delight.

Except, of course, when it came to the idea of his *mother* having sex. Throughout elementary school, Nate would size up the men we came into contact with—fathers of his classmates, the guys who worked at the pizza place or the corner deli, random passersby.

"He likes you," Nate would say to me from time to time, his eyes narrowing at the offending party. I sometimes got a similar vibe. It was disconcerting that Nate could feel it, too.

"I DON'T KNOW WHERE to begin," I say to Mitchell a few days after I return from Houston. I reach for a tissue. There is something pathetic about crying within the first minute of a therapy session, but it's better than the other extreme. On days when I leave Mitchell's office and feel the beginnings of a migraine thrumming at my temples, I know I haven't gone deep enough during my session—and wasted two hundred dollars to boot.

"Let's just sit for a moment. You can start with whatever rises to the surface."

I find this approach soothing. Once I still the chatter in my brain, there is no question of what is weighing most heavily on me. Daniel's face appears before me; his voice sounds in my ears. I tell Mitchell about Daniel's discovery.

"Do you think I'm screwing up my kid?" I say, wiping at my tears. This is my biggest fear. More than anything in this world, I want to be a good mother.

"Molly," Mitchell says without missing a beat, "I think you're screwing him up the exact average amount."

I laugh, and before I can control it, my brain pivots—to my mother, to Jim, to Mahikari. Did my mother screw *me* up the exact average amount, too?

IT'S SPRING, 1983. I am ten years old, and the horrors of sixth grade are coming to an end. The age difference between my classmates and me means more now than it did when I was eight, when the decision was made to skip a grade. In middle school, girls wear bras, talk about boys, get their periods. This world is not mine.

I'm too embarrassed to ask my mother to buy me a bra I don't really need. I can't talk to her about how badly I want my period, either. What my mother and I do talk about is the same thing she talks about with Jim: Mahikari.

Ever since third grade, I've been sick all the time. Head colds, pink eye, and strep throat are my top three maladies. But Mahikari, where my mother turns for all her wisdom, teaches that illness is a cleansing, that nothing should interrupt the outward flow of toxins. And so, instead of medicine, my mother gives me light.

She holds her hand above my forehead while I close my eyes and listen to the sound of her chanting in a language neither of us understands. I am the only one in our family who willingly lets her do this. My father calls Mahikari "macaroni." My sister is outwardly hostile about most things related to my mother, and especially Mahikari.

I, however, am a good girl.

Several times a week, I sit before her in the required position: kneeling on the floor with my back straight, feet tucked under my body, left big toe over right, left thumb over right, a prayer in front of my heart. We bow to each other, and I close my eyes. She claps three times and begins to chant: *"Goku bi JI-so gen gen shikari . . ."*

I sit, sensing my mother's open palm in front of my forehead until her voice booms, *"O-shizu-mari!,"* releasing my spirit from the hold of the light.

Now that I'm ten, my mother tells me, I'm old enough to join.

"Would you like to take *kenshu*?" my mother asks, using the official term for Mahikari's first initiation.

I see the hopeful expectation in my mother's eyes. Jim is moving to New York, so she won't have anyone to give her light. My mom needs me.

"You would make me the happiest mother in the world," she adds.

Mahikari is for adults. It's boring and weird, but my mom's suggestion that I could do something so grown-up makes me feel important, special. How can I pass up an opportunity to bring my mother joy?

"Okay," I say, not understanding exactly what I'm agreeing to.

In the photograph taken at my *kenshu* ceremony, I'm seated in the first row. I look very small. I'm wearing my nicest clothes, a pastel collared blouse and a khaki skirt. My socks are pulled up to my knees, and, according to Japanese custom, I, like everyone else, am shoeless. My long hair, a light sandy color I hardly remember, is parted in the middle and pinned back with two barrettes. I am unsmiling, serious, in sharp contrast with my mother, who stands behind me, beaming.

"I NEVER REALLY THOUGHT about it before," I say to Mitchell now, anger bubbling up to the edges of my awareness. I'm starting to connect the dots, and the picture they form is disturbing. "But Jim is the whole reason my mom got into Mahikari in the first place. And it was pretty fucked up for her to ask me to join a cult. Not that she'd ever call it a cult. But no medicine? And all that money they asked for? How could she indoctrinate a ten-year-old with that crap? I mean, I was Nate's age!"

Mitchell looks at me sympathetically. "It's very common for people to remember, or even relive, childhood experiences when their own children are at that same age."

I nod, picturing my small, sickly ten-year-old self standing shoulder to shoulder with Nate. I feel a surge of protectiveness for this younger me, amplified by pointless outrage. It all happened over thirty years ago. "But what should I *do* with all this?"

Mitchell raises his eyes. His fingers form two flying buttresses over his mouth, supporting his words until they're ready to come out.

"What you do with it is up to you, Molly," he begins. "It sounds like you're angry at your mother for involving you in what was supposed to be *her* journey."

"I *am* angry," I say. It feels good to acknowledge the truth of this, even if I can't imagine telling my mother how I feel. I think of the wounded expression she wears when my sister gets angry at her. I never want to be the cause of that look.

"And then there are your fears about how *your* journey into open marriage is impacting your own children."

I nod again, and whatever rage I've mustered melts into guilt.

"Take a minute to feel what you're feeling, Molly," Mitchell says gently. "You're in rich terrain right now."

I try. Images stampede through my mind, each of them kicking up emotional dust. Me—my throat on fire with untreated infections, and again, so serious in the *kenshu* photograph. Jim at the dinner table, making my mother laugh. Daniel, reading the words *open marriage* on Stewart's laptop. Nate, looking sideways at the men who smile at me.

Later, when I stand to go, Mitchell says, "You've shown yourself to be a pretty resilient person, Molly." His smile turns wry, and he answers the question I haven't asked aloud. "For the record, I think your mother screwed *you* up the average amount, too."

FOR THE NEXT FEW weeks, Daniel is consumed with my whereabouts.

"Where are you going?" he asks me. "Are you *really* going to Jessie's? Are you *sure* you're going to the gym?" Stewart, meanwhile, continues to come and go as he pleases, without Daniel giving him a second glance. I feel guilty and furious at the same time, and vent both feelings to Stew.

"Why doesn't Daniel ask where *you're* going?" I shout without shouting, late one night behind the closed door of our bedroom. "Why doesn't anyone seem to care if fathers have sex, but every mother is supposed to be the goddamn Virgin Mary?"

"Maybe you should take it as a compliment," Stew says. "He needs you more than he needs me. Or maybe he's worried about you."

"Neither of those possibilities makes me feel any better."

"How about if I sit Daniel down for a little man-to-man?"

"What will you say to him?" I ask.

"Leave that to me," says Stewart.

It takes all my willpower to refrain from eavesdropping. I know both parties well enough to be sure neither will ever disclose the full contents of their conversation. Afterward, Stew tells me it went fine. And Daniel asks to talk to me.

"I'm sorry I've been asking where you're going all the time, Mom," he begins. "I know it's private. And it's not fair that I never give Dad the third degree."

"It's okay, honey," I answer, marveling, as I've done for years, at the cosmic maturity of this kid. "It's just that, I don't think you actually want to know if I'm out on a date. And sometimes I really am just going to Jessie's or to the gym."

"Yeah," he says pensively. "Could you just lie to me? I'll try not to ask where you're going, but if I do, can you just lie if you have a date?"

This, of course, is what I've been doing all along. But having his permission, his acknowledgment that my lies are in his best interest, eases a bit of the guilt my dishonesty has produced. Yet plenty of shame remains.

THE NEXT TIME I see Leo is after a long hiatus. He's been on a sailing trip with friends, from New York to Canadian waters. During his weeks away, he sends photographs of himself, standing on the boat, suntanned and windblown, or mugging in front of a kitschy sign in a picturesque harbor town. He sends me vague invitations by email: *Someday you should come along for a sail—with your guitar!*

The day after his return, Leo texts in the early afternoon, all but begging me to come over. But begging isn't necessary. The kids are at school and a midday booty call without Daniel's questioning gaze is just what the doctor ordered.

I shower quickly and take the subway uptown. As I walk from the station to Leo's apartment, I try to catch a glimpse of myself in storefront windows and side-view mirrors—checking my nose for boogers, hoping that the sweat collecting at my hairline isn't making my foundation run. Leo greets me at the door, half-dressed as usual, and through a joint effort, we are both naked in under a minute. But then it stops feeling familiar.

I suppose there's a reason why sailors have the reputation they do, being out at sea for long stretches without access to women. Sex is consensual that day, but it is also rough—rougher than it's ever been before, and rougher than I want it to be. I give myself over to his desires and try to squelch my own. Leo bites my lip, hard, leaving a bruise like smudged lipstick that I can feel for days. And once the sex is over, our pillow talk, something we typically linger over, is cut short. He has so much to do. He thanks me for coming over on such short notice. And then he ushers me out the door.

Even as I walk back to the train, I question my memory of what just happened. But the pain on my lip won't let me lie to myself.

Why didn't I stop him? Why couldn't I tell him how he was making me feel—like a Grubhub delivery to a ravenous man, devoured without even the civility of napkins or utensils? Because, really, who am I? I am not special. I am not loved. I'm not even Leo's mistress. I am his piece of ass on the side. What did I expect anyway?

"I FEEL LIKE SHIT," I say to Mitchell the next week. "I thought freedom was supposed to be fun."

"Nothing is fun all the time," Mitchell answers. The reasonableness of this statement makes me sigh. "Let's get more specific about your feelings. 'Like shit' is a bit vague."

"Okay," I say. "How about out of control? It's like I'm just reacting to what men want. I'm not asserting myself at all. And getting attention, having sex—it feels good but it's so temporary. Then afterward, I feel like shit. Sorry—I mean, afterward, I feel empty."

The act of saying the word brings the feeling to the surface. Empty. I feel empty. I reach for a tissue as the tears start to flow.

Mitchell pauses as I cry, looking at the ceiling, as is his habit when he contemplates what to say next. "Molly, let me ask you something. What's the *opposite* of that feeling, of being empty?"

"The opposite?" I say. "I guess filled up?"

"Great," says Mitchell. "So let's veer away for a moment from the things you're doing that bring about an empty feeling. Instead, I'd like you to frame this differently. Can you remember some moments recently when you felt filled up?"

I stop and think. When *do* I feel filled up? I think of my conversations with Daniel, reading stories to Nate in bed, letting myself be held by Stewart.

"I'm filled up by my kids," I say. "And also by Stewart. But it's weird. Giving them too much of myself also makes me feel empty. Or maybe I'll just feel empty no matter what I do." This thought threatens to create a new batch of tears, and I grab another tissue.

"Hmm," says Mitchell, creasing his eyes with concentration. "An idea is coming to me, and I wonder if it will be helpful."

I look at him expectantly.

"I think there's a hole in your bucket."

A hole in my bucket. I nod. I like the concreteness of the image.

"You're filling up with all the good things in your life, including your husband and children," he continues, "but then they drain out the bottom and you feel empty again. You've got to patch the hole so the good things don't leak away."

"How do I do that?"

"That's the work," says Mitchell. "That's what you need to figure out."

OVER THE NEXT FEW weeks, I think about my bucket, the insidious hole.

One night, I watch Stewart sleep, his lips puffing air, touching the borders of a snore. From my vantage point, it seems like Stew is having nothing but fun as he jaunts along the open-marriage path.

What am I doing wrong? Why is his bucket in such better shape than my own? An old folk song loops through my head, a plaintive whine:

With what shall I fix it, dear Stewart, with what?

First, I decide not to see Leo again. Although I can't feel the bruise on my lip anymore, it lingers in my memory, reminding me of how self-esteem gushed from my bucket the last time I slept with him, the degradation I felt. As if to confirm my feeling that Leo doesn't really care about me, he stops texting. I fight the urge to send him a message. It seems absurd to initiate contact just to say I don't want to see him anymore. His silence has made its own declaration.

And then there's Laurent. We've graduated to a new level of seediness—and I'm not sure if it's higher or lower than bar bathrooms, Breather spaces, and my cubicle at Greendesk.

The Liberty Inn—a beacon to sexual freedom itself—is the sole occupant of a triangle of land in a rarely visited corner of Manhattan. One might pass it by taking a detour around the West Side Highway entrance at 14th Street, maybe while making a delivery to one of the warehouses of the Meatpacking District. The Liberty Inn is available for either two- or three-hour bookings. Cash payment is preferred, and Laurent is willing to fork over a few twenties as long as he doesn't have to use a credit card. Some of the rooms have mirrors on the ceilings. The furniture is covered in easy-to-wipe plastic so the only bodily fluids a couple encounters are their own. The front desk will even call the room ten minutes before time runs out—less of a *wake up* than a *get out* courtesy call. The depressed-looking housekeeping staff—with whom I avoid eye contact—has to ready the room for the next patrons.

The Liberty Inn has become Laurent's and my special place.

One night, as we scurry like cockroaches to gather our stuff before the paid hours are up and we're charged a late fee, I screw up my courage to make a pronouncement. It comes out in the form of a question.

"Do you think we could go somewhere else next time?" I ask, looking for my bra, which Laurent briefly used to tie my hands together before flinging it away. "This place is just so . . . I don't know . . . skeezy."

The space between Laurent's eyebrows contracts. "What iz theez word?"

"*Skeezy*? It's like 'disgusting.' 'Gross.' Just look at this place and you can figure out the definition yourself," I say.

"I theenk it eez *sexy*," says Laurent, coming up behind me to cup my breasts as I spot my bra under the air conditioner. "Like you." He kisses me on the neck.

I bat him away. "We only have three minutes to get out of here."

"Okay, okay," he says, holding up his hands and smiling like a little boy caught stealing from his mother's purse.

I pull my dress over my head and step into my sandals. We run down the stairs and hand our key through the opening in the bullet-proof glass. The front-desk clerk grunts and buzzes us through the two sets of doors that lead to the street. Outside, the winds of 14th Street, 10th Avenue, and the West Side Highway have created a vortex of garbage. Plastic grocery bags and fast-food containers swirl in the air with the first leaves of fall.

"I mean, look at this place," I say again. "Skeezy."

Laurent takes my hand and pulls me along 14th Street. There are never any taxis so far west, especially at this time of night. "You make zee point," he says. "We weel go zumplace new zee next time. I want to ask you to go weez me anyway."

"Really?" I say, perking up. "Where?"

He wraps his arm around my shoulders to keep me in step with his stride as he whispers into my ear: "Eet eez a sex club . . ."

I duck out from under his arm and stop walking. "Wait a

second," I say. "I told you about the times I went to Le Trapeze with Stewart. I'm not going back there."

"Joost relax," he says. "It eez a different place. In zee Bowery. I promise, you weel love it."

When I get home, I pay the babysitter and head straight for my computer. I type *Bowery sex club* into the search bar, and up pops an article from *Time Out New York* published in 2013. I begin to read:

> *I imagine that there are many good reasons why you should never attend a swingers' club. With the opening of Bowery Bliss—a 4,000-square-foot, multilevel sexploratorium at the nexus of the Lower East Side, Chinatown and Nolita—an unfashionable location need not be one of them.*

The more I read, the more my Le Trapeze PTSD flares. No matter if I said I liked it at the time. No matter that I ended up going more than once. Le Trapeze was not my cup of tea, and Bowery Bliss, despite its classy locale, doesn't seem to be any better.

I decide to rip the Band-Aid off right away. I climb into bed and send Laurent a text: *I looked up some info on Bowery Bliss. Sorry, but group sex just isn't for me. Let's go to a nice hotel for once, okay?*

Laurent sends back a single emoji. Pouty face.

I've seen that face before. In person. I think of all the pushback Laurent gave me about wearing a condom, how he complained about the discomfort, said it was like having sex with a rubber glove, told me he needed to feel me, all of me, in order to orgasm. And then I think with shame about how I eventually relented, and how I rationalized this choice: *He's going to take his condom off anyway,* I thought. *I'm on the pill. I'll ask him to come only when we're having anal sex.* (I'd graduated from butt plugs months ago.) *I'll just keep getting tested for STDs.*

And now Laurent is asking me to relent again. To turn my back on a decision I made long ago: to never go to a sex club again.

I wish Stewart were here. I can't remember if he's out with another woman, or working late, or getting a drink with friends. I wish I could run this by him, ask him what I should do. But then a certainty rears its head from someplace deep inside me. I don't need Stew's advice. I can't go to another sex club. I won't do it.

As if reading my mind, Laurent writes again: *Just one time. I promise.*

Sorry, Laurent. (Why am I apologizing?) *I've made my decision. No more sex clubs.*

I wait as the three little dots transform into a message.

So my pleasure is unimportant to you? he writes. Another pouty face. Something inside me snaps.

What the fuck?! Everything I do is for your pleasure! Stop being such an immature asshole.

My heart beats inside my throat as the three dots blink for an eternity.

Very well. Perhaps it is time I look for another button.

I stare dumbly at his message. I remember something he said to me on our first date. When I made an oblique reference to his wife—*does she suspect?*—he avoided the question. Instead, he relayed something his Argentine mother used to say to him: *Women are like buttons. If you lose one, you can always find another.* Why hadn't I run in the other direction?

A wave of nausea sweeps over me. He's trying to pressure me into following his every whim, trying to make me feel guilty about all the ways in which I'm *not* pleasing him. Do what he wants, or watch him find someone who will.

I picture the hole in my bucket, and I can almost see my self-worth spilling onto the floor. I have to stanch the flow, and suddenly I know how.

Go ahead, I write back. *You and I are done.*

I hit Send. And before I can see his manipulative or cruel reply—or, worse, no reply at all—I block his number on my phone.

Then I lie facedown on my pillow. A shred of dignity waves like a lone blade of grass in an otherwise empty field. I've let go of Leo. I've dismissed Laurent. But it's not either of them that I want right now.

I want Stewart. I need Stewart.

I hear a keening wail. I hear it before I realize the sound is coming from me. I bury my head under every pillow within reach. I can't control the volume of the sobs, so I muffle them instead, trying to cushion their force as they tear through my body. I cry for so long that I don't remember stopping. I fall asleep with the lights on, my head still buried in pillows soaked in my tears and stiffening with dried snot, my eyes swollen, my face a map of broken blood vessels.

And when he gets home, this is how Stewart finds me.

CHAPTER 10

"SO. LET'S GET STARTED. Why are you here?"

It's a straightforward question posed by our new couples therapist, Evelyn—a matronly woman with a silver no-fuss bob, a large jade pendant hanging between the mounds of her prodigious bosom. But answering it is overwhelming.

Stewart makes a sweeping gesture toward me, as in *Go right ahead. Tell the nice lady why we're here.* Counseling was my idea—or, to be more accurate, my ultimatum.

It's been two weeks since my "breakdown," as I like to call it. There's something comforting about the word, something alluring about a full collapse. In fact, I am using every bit of force I can muster to keep up the illusion of functionality to my children, to the outside world. Stewart, however, is privy to the truth, and this is important to me. He needs to know that I'm wrecked. Finished. Kaput.

Evelyn comes highly recommended by Mitchell, but I can't make myself feel hopeful. Perhaps the problem is the cavernous space we now occupy, more than triple the square footage of Mitchell's cozy office. Stewart feels far away on Evelyn's too-wide couch. And Evelyn herself is inaccessible across the expanse of an oversized coffee table.

I take a deep breath. "We're here because I don't want to be in an open marriage anymore. But Stewart does."

Stew sighs heavily, and Evelyn nods toward him.

"You disagree with that, Stewart?"

He looks at me sideways, an accusation in his eyes. I look back innocently. I know I've oversimplified, but there's also truth in what I've said.

"It's not that I want to keep the marriage open regardless of how Molly feels. It's that I know she's going to change her mind." He turns and faces me. "You're unhappy right now, I get it. But you have to give it time. You'll meet somebody new and you'll feel differently."

Tears sting my eyes. We haven't even been here five minutes. "I don't want somebody new," I say. "I want *you*."

"Oh, baby," says Stewart. "You have me. You'll *always* have me."

"It doesn't feel that way. I feel so alone."

"You're not alone, Molly!" he shouts, exasperated. "I'm here next to you! Right now!"

Evelyn raises her hand to stop him, the gesture of a school crossing guard. It does seem like we're back in elementary school, relying on the grown-up to check both ways for danger, to guide us safely through this crossroads.

"Stewart, what Molly has said is that she *feels* alone. Feelings aren't facts, so it's better not to try to dispute a feeling."

Stew holds up two hands and bows his head. Whether this is a sarcastic or a sincere mea culpa, I can't determine.

"Molly," Evelyn continues, "can you get more specific about what you need from Stewart to not feel alone?"

"I want him to be happy when he's home," I say.

"You can't force me to be happy, Molly!" Stewart erupts. "Sorry. I'm not supposed to talk."

"No, it's okay for you to talk," says Evelyn. "And your point is well taken. We'll come back later to the question of your happiness. Try again, Molly. What do *you* need to feel less alone?"

I think about it. My loneliness is erratic. I try to climb inside the feeling and figure out what I truly need.

"I need to have more fun with Stewart," I say. "We used to have so much fun."

"Okay," says Evelyn, nodding encouragingly. "And what would having fun with Stewart look like? What would the two of you do?" I open my mouth to answer, but she says, "Don't tell me. Tell Stewart."

I turn to face him. "I want you to take me to breakfast. Last week you took Beth out for breakfast, and it hurt my feelings because you and I never do that anymore. And I love breakfast."

Stewart laughs. "You certainly do," he says, reaching for my hand. "I will absolutely take you out for breakfast this week."

"You will?" I say, brightening.

"Of course!" he answers. "Pick a day when you don't have any workshops or meetings and we'll go while the kids are at school. Is that it?"

My shoulders slump as I consider his words. "Well, now I feel like you're just checking an item off a list. I want you to *want* to go to breakfast with me. And for it to be *your* idea."

Stew drops my hand. He throws himself backward against the couch with enough force that I bounce a little.

"I can't win!" he shouts, addressing Evelyn now. "No matter what I do, she gets upset!"

"Okay, let's try something else," says Evelyn. "We're going to do a listening exercise. Stewart, you're going to tell Molly why you feel like you can't win. Molly, you're going to repeat back to Stewart everything he says to you. You don't have to repeat his words verbatim, but you can't editorialize or present your own position. I'll be here to help. Go ahead, Stew. Look at Molly. Start with what you just said, 'I feel like I can't win. No matter what I do, you get upset.'"

Stewart rubs his hand over his face and turns to me. I can see reluctance written there. But he does as he's told.

"I feel like I can't win," he says. "No matter what I do, you get upset."

"Now you repeat that back," says Evelyn, addressing me.

"You feel like you can't win," I say. "No matter what you do, I get upset."

"Did she get that right, Stewart?" asks Evelyn.

"Yup."

"Okay, let's keep going. What else?"

"You want me to read your mind," Stew says. "And if I don't guess what you're thinking, you're disappointed in me."

"I want you to read my mind," I say. "And if you can't guess what I'm thinking, I act like I'm disappointed in you."

"Right," says Stewart. I watch the muscles in his face relax. I'm feeling more relaxed, too.

"How does this feel, Stewart?" asks Evelyn. "To have Molly really hear what you're saying?"

"It feels good! It's like having my own little parrot!"

I hit him lightly on the arm, and he squeezes my knee.

Evelyn beams at us. Hope starts to rise within me again.

We continue our Molly-Wants-a-Cracker Exercise, as Stew calls it, and then switch roles. When the hour is up, we're both laughing.

"I want the two of you to practice this technique at home. And remember, Molly, it's okay to need Stewart, and to tell him what you need—whether you decide to keep the marriage open or not." This concept hits me with an unexpected blast of relief. Our marriage—whether it's monogamous or not—needs attention and care. And we can work on it without having to make any final decisions about staying open.

"Next time, Stewart," she continues, "we'll talk about what *you* need from Molly to feel happier in your marriage. Give it some thought."

As Stew and I descend in the elevator together, I ask him, "So what do you think of her?"

"I liked her more than I thought I would," he admits. "What about you?"

"I think she was helpful." The doors open and we're in the lobby. Stewart heads toward the exit, in a palpable hurry to get back to work, to take a breather from all this touchy-feely talk. But I don't want to let go of the closeness I felt, sitting beside him on the too-big couch—not yet. I'm feeling generous. I want to give him something. "What's the name of that dating site again? The one that's good for people in open relationships—the one that chick Kathy told you about?"

"You mean Katie?" He knows how much I enjoy confusing the names of the women he dates. "It's called OkCupid. Yeah, it seems cool. You can even choose 'non-monogamous' as your status."

"Right. I think I'll start an account. I mean, if you agree to keep seeing Evelyn with me, I'll stop dating shitty men from Ashley Madison and give this open-marriage thing a real try."

"That's great, baby," says Stew, holding me by the shoulders and locking his eyes on mine. I love it when he does this. When he makes me feel this seen. "Thank you for that." He kisses me lightly on the lips. "I gotta run to work—but I'll be home on the early side."

I resist asking him what "early" means.

THAT NIGHT, I DELETE my Ashley Madison account and sign up on OkCupid. There it is. *Non-monogamous* is in the drop-down menu, nestled among *Single, Seeing Someone,* and *It's Complicated.* But it all seems complicated to me.

In my OkCupid profile, my name is Molly, not Mercedes. I select a photo of myself that reveals my face. I start answering questions that will help me find my ideal match. Half of them are redundant, as if the algorithm is unconvinced that I understand what "non-monogamous" means.

> *How willing are you to date someone who has another partner?*
> *If your partner told you they had kissed someone else, how would you react?*
> *How important to you is exclusivity in a relationship?*

I choose among the nuance-free answers provided: *Very willing. I'd be fine with it. Not important.* And just like that, I'm officially in an open marriage.

For the next few days, my OkCupid account becomes the center of my universe. I soon learn how this "free" dating site makes money. Unless I buy a Premium membership, I can't even read the messages in my inbox. I upgrade and start the epic task of sorting wheat from chaff. But once I figure out how to filter for men who are also in open relationships, my pool of prospective partners dwindles from 537 to 12. And my top match—which is reassuring, I suppose—is Stewart.

"What the hell?" I say to him late one night as we lean against the kitchen island and I show him his own profile on my phone. "I thought you said this was the best app for people in open marriages."

"Well, they added the 'non-monogamous' option pretty recently. I like it because I don't have to explain myself over and over again. But don't limit yourself to men who are also open. How about the single guys?"

"Yeah, I guess so. But I also want to learn about this whole non-monogamous world, you know?" I scroll down and pause. "Like, what's up with this guy? Liam. He says he's non-monogamous but also single. What does that even mean?"

Stew looks over my shoulder at the person in question. The photo shows an athletic, outdoorsy type with a full head of light brown hair, dreamy blue eyes, sensual lips. He reads aloud the highlights from Liam's profile. "A hetero-flexible sommelier who is more than ten years younger than you. Go for it, baby. What do you have to lose?"

LIAM LIVES IN QUEENS, which may as well be Philadelphia in terms of its public transportation links to Park Slope. We decide to meet at a park on the Lower East Side, not far from the restaurant where he works. I arrive first and perch on a bench while I glance around, trying to spot him and look casual at the same time. For a man who makes his living in wine, he's arranged for a date that's unsettlingly alcohol-free.

A good-looking guy in skinny jeans walks toward me across the patchy grass. He is coatless in the chilly fall air, a linen shirt unbuttoned enough to expose his hairless chest. As he comes closer, I see a face that is the picture of contentment, too relaxed to be disturbed by smiling.

"Molly," he says without a question mark. He opens his arms during his last few strides, and I stand to be engulfed in a full-body hug, which feels too intimate for a first meeting yet devoid of sexual undertones. "It's so, so good to meet you," he says into my neck.

"You too," I reply, blushing.

"Tell me about yourself," he says, sitting close to me on the bench. His leg is touching mine, but it doesn't feel like a come-on. Nevertheless, I'm having trouble absorbing the force of his eye contact. "How long have you been polyamorous?"

"What?" I stammer, shaken by the word. "Oh. I'm in an open

marriage, but I'm not sure if I'm polyamorous at all. Or maybe I just don't like the label." I blush more deeply as I realize I might have insulted him. "I mean, not that there's anything wrong with it. Oh God. Sorry. I sound like George Costanza."

"That's cool," says Liam mildly. He probably doesn't even get the reference. He must have been nine years old when *Seinfeld* aired. "Polyamory is still very misunderstood. Even the poly community can't agree on what it is."

"Really?" I say. "Because I could certainly use a tutorial!"

Liam doesn't exactly laugh. It's more like a Zen smile that evokes the *sense* of laughter. "In that case, I'm your guy. My mother was poly, and I was raised in a poly commune. In Northern California," he adds unnecessarily.

"Wow. My parents were in an open marriage, too, but they won't even use that term. My mother says she had 'an affair' with my father's blessing."

"Uh-huh," he says. He must be the first person I've met who's unfazed by this disclosure. "People can get really hung up on language, you know? Like, some purists don't consider open marriage to be polyamory at all. They think it's too hierarchical—since spouses are automatically 'primary' and other partners are 'secondary' or whatever."

"What about you?" I ask.

"Well, I'm solo poly," he answers.

"What does that mean?" It sounds like an oxymoron to me, but I'm trying to keep an open mind.

"It means I'm my own primary relationship. So I don't intend to get married, or even for my romantic relationships to last forever. But that doesn't mean I don't take relationships seriously." I don't doubt him. He's looking at me with a steadiness that can only be described as, well, serious. "It's like having more than one close friend—people love their friends, but they don't need a legal document forcing them to commit to their friends for life. And nobody would say, 'I can't believe you've been seeing other friends.' You know what I mean?"

I nod, feeling excitement bubble up within me as I take in this idea. "Yeah, I know exactly what you mean." I think of Edie. Nina. Kayla. Jessie. Each of them fills a different role in my life. And I wouldn't want to part with any of them. Why couldn't it be that way in the realm of sex and romance?

"I've also met some of my partners through other partners," he continues. "That's the best. When you love two people who also love each other."

At this, the bubble of excitement starts to deflate. I try to conjure "love" for one of Stewart's girlfriends. All that comes is a heavy feeling akin to dread.

Liam reads my reaction with disquieting accuracy. "So I'm guessing you haven't experienced compersion yet?" he asks.

"Com-what?"

"*Compersion.* It's a positive feeling you get when your partner is with someone else. Kind of like the opposite of jealousy."

"No," I say quickly. "Definitely haven't experienced that one."

Liam's face wears the expression of a teacher who realizes his pupil needs serious remediation. "There's a book you ought to read," he says.

On my way home, I stop by the Strand—a bookstore large enough to contain the embarrassment I feel at picking up a copy of *The Ethical Slut: A Practical Guide to Polyamory, Open Relationships & Other Adventures.* According to Liam, this is the bible of polyamory. He's told me that I'll find *compersion* in the index, and sure enough, there it is—sandwiched between *communication* and *compassion* on one side and *competitiveness* and *conflict* on the other.

On the F train, I turn to chapter 18 and read: "Some polyfolk use the word 'compersion' to describe the feeling of joy that comes from seeing your partner sexually happy with someone else."

I shut the book. I think I'd better start on page 1.

A FEW DAYS LATER, Liam sends me a text, inviting me to hang out at the bar of the restaurant where he works.

Late shift every night this week—come by and I'll keep you in drinks.

Without a set day or time to meet, I feel lost in terms of when to show up. I decide a weekday is good. If I wait until the kids are in bed and Stew is home from work, I'll arrive late enough—late enough for what, I can't say.

I walk through the double doors at ten thirty on a Tuesday night and am shocked to see the place is packed. Don't these people have jobs? I also note that rather than Liam, there's a woman behind the bar. A young, beautiful, impossibly fashionable woman who appears to be made of sunshine and stardust.

I wedge my way through the crowd and slide onto the last remaining stool. I focus on looking purposeful. It takes several tries to hang my bag on the hook at my knees, and once I've managed that, I fidget to smooth my skirt under my butt. All the while, I keep darting my eyes at the bartender, wondering with a growing sense of panic how to explain who I am, the cosmic glitch of my existence in this place of soft techno tracks and softer blue light. When she looks up, I flag her over, still unsure of which words will come out.

"Hi there," she says. "How ya doin' tonight?" She's even prettier up close—carelessly tousled hair, a button nose, huge turquoise eyes, and a voice that matches Liam's California lilt. Their hiring policy must be posted like the rules for riding a roller coaster: *You Must Be This Gorgeous to Work Here.*

"I'm good, good," I say, feeling extraordinarily foolish and out of place. "I'm, um, a friend of Liam's. He said he'd be here tonight?"

"Oh cool, cool." Is she teasing me by echoing my phrasing? Or just trying to make me feel like *less* of an idiot? I'm so consumed by analyzing this first exchange that I almost miss what she says next: "You must be Molly. Liam told me to keep an eye out for you. I'll let him know you're here. What can I get you in the meantime?"

Even though Liam invited me, I'm stunned to be expected. "Great, great," I say in my addled way, losing any scrap of confidence I've gained. "I'll take a glass of the house white."

"We can do better than that," she says, laughing. "Liam will kill me if I give a friend of his house wine."

I'm on my second glass of a "bright Viognier"—a wine I've never heard of and whose name I wouldn't dare attempt to pronounce aloud—when I smell Liam's grassy cologne.

"Hey, you," he says, placing a hand on the small of my back and kissing my cheek. His five-o'clock shadow is as nice to feel and inhale as it is to look at.

"Hi!" I say too loudly. I'm like a warthog that got into the gazelle pen at the zoo. But the gazelles don't seem to notice.

Liam reaches over to take a sip of my wine and nods his approval. "I see Thea is taking good care of you," he says. "I'll ask the kitchen to send over our roasted carrot soup. It pairs nicely with this one."

"That sounds amazing. Thanks," I say. I'm starving, but it looks like I'm grazing à la gazelle tonight.

He leans in again, and I get another whiff of his scent. Maybe I can subsist on the smell of him alone. "I can get away for a break in about half an hour," he whispers into my ear. "Can you hang out until then?"

I nod mutely, and he kisses my cheek again, this time catching the corner of my mouth.

When I've finished my third glass of wine, as well as my soup—which, thankfully, was garnished with a smattering of fortifying chickpeas—Liam reappears behind me. He reaches under the bar, stroking my leg and grabbing my bag from its hook with an easy motion that registers in my groin. His other hand takes mine and leads me outside.

I follow him to a shadowy spot between the door and the bay windows and wonder how many other women he has brought here. I also wonder if a chickpea is stuck in my teeth. But when he leans down from his perfect height and kisses me, these questions don't seem to matter much. His kiss is confident but gentle, commanding but respectful—the Sensitive Leading Man in real life. One kiss blends into the next, and I lose all sense of time. Making out with Liam is a multisensory experience. The touch of his soft lips, his grassy scent, the taste of his tongue, as if he's been chewing on organic mint leaves all night, and perhaps he has. Even the hum of traffic and the wafts of conversation from passersby seem to emanate from Liam himself, the conductor of this soundscape.

"Get home safely, Molly," he says finally, and I open my eyes to meet his. The polyamory in his gaze is as evident as the California in his voice. This is a man who is not afraid to fall in love.

HEY THERE, Liam texts the next day. *Thanks for stopping by last night. It was great 2 C U.*

I try to submerge my visceral reaction to text-speak and focus on the memory of Liam's soft lips and sexy stubble.

It was great seeing you too, I write back. *Thanks for all the free drinks!*

Anytime. BTW, have you ever been 2 Poly Cocktails? HMU if you want to go! Next one is Monday night.

Okay, thanks. I'll let you know!

Right after googling *What does HMU mean in a text?,* I type *Poly Cocktails* into the search bar. It's exactly what it sounds like.

"Poly Cocktails," the website states, "was started on Valentine's Day 2007 by three polyamorous activists and friends as a way to create a social outlet for the local poly community in New York." I scan the navigation bar and click next on "What is Polyamory?"

> *Polyamory (derived from the Greek and Latin roots for "many loves") is also known as Ethical or Consensual Non-Monogamy (ENM or CNM). In a polyamorous relationship, people can have meaningful emotional and/or physical relationships with multiple people simultaneously, with the full knowledge and consent of everyone involved.*

So far so good. Nothing new or shocking here. I read on:

> *There are as many forms of polyamory as there are people who practice it, but the main hallmarks are honesty, constant communication and emotional openness. In fact, many of the lessons learned from polyamory are applicable to traditional relationships as well. While there may be some overlap, polyamory is NOT the same as swinging, spouse swapping, or kink play. Polyamory does not imply any particular sexual behavior or rules; rather, it encourages people to explore and define their own rules in a way that makes sense to them and respects the needs and desires of all parties involved.*

All of that works for me, I think. Constant communication? Emotional openness? No pressure to do anything you don't want to do? Who could argue with that?

THE NEXT NIGHT, STEWART and I are grabbing an early dinner at MooBurger before Nate's school play. Families spill out of every booth. Haggard parents urge children to take bites while attempting to converse over the chaotic din.

"Why did you pick this place again?" asks Stew as he moves his chair to make way for a stroller.

Our own kids aren't with us. Nate is eating pizza with the cast, and Daniel, now an eighth grader, is hanging out with friends and will meet us at the play. My children's growing independence is simultaneously thrilling and horrifying. *O, glorious freedom!* shouts one part of me. *O, death of purpose!* grieves another.

"Sorry. I guess it's just force of habit. This is my go-to place near school. Plus they have gluten-free buns and wine!" I gesture happily at the spread in front of me.

"Yeah," says Stew. "But they don't have whiskey. Or even real soda. I hate that Boylan crap." He takes a begrudging sip of water.

"Do you want to order a beer?" I suggest guiltily. If he brought me to a place without a wine list, I'd be sure to complain. He shakes his head, and I think of a way to change the subject. "Have you heard of Poly Cocktails?"

Stewart looks at me sideways. "Um, yes?"

"Why the question mark?" I ask, reaching for one of his fries. "You've either heard of it or you haven't."

"What I'm questioning is whether you really want to know," he says. "How can I put this? You tend to ask questions and then get angry when I answer honestly."

"You're totally right," I say. He looks at me with surprise.

"I am? I thought you'd deny that till your dying day."

"I'm working on it, okay? I seem to have enrolled in Polyamory 101 with Liam. He's the one who invited me to Poly Cocktails. And he told me about something called *compersion*. Have you heard of that, too?"

"Yeah," says Stew, laughing. "I'm taking the same course, but I think I'm about two weeks ahead of you in the syllabus."

I grip my wineglass with both hands. So Stewart is dating someone who's teaching him the same concepts I'm learning from Liam. This is a good thing, right? Getting us on the same page? Then why do I feel consumed by jealousy? I try to remember my new *Ethical Slut* wisdom: "Jealousy is often the mask worn by the most difficult inner conflict you have going on right now."

"Just go slowly for me, okay? Did you actually go to Poly Cocktails with someone?"

"Not exactly," he says. "But I did go on a date . . . kind of . . . with someone who attends regularly. I doubt I'll see her again, though."

At this, my body starts to relax. *See? Nothing to feel jealous of here,* I tell myself. "Is she someone you've told me about?"

"Nope," says Stew. "I knew you'd make fun of me if I did. Right before you got upset."

"Why are you so sure I'll get upset?" I ask, starting to get upset.

"Fine," he says, signaling the waitress for our check. "I'll tell you, but only because we have to leave for the play soon. I like to have an escape hatch."

"Okay. You have five minutes. I promise not to interrupt."

"I can do it in less than two," Stew says. "I met this woman named Tinkerbell on OkCupid, and—"

"Tinkerbell?!" I interrupt—loudly. "That's her actual *name*?" Stew stays silent and raises his eyebrows at me.

"Sorry. I'll be quiet. Go on."

"As I was saying," Stewart says, handing his credit card to the waitress, "the name she goes by on OKC is Tinkerbell, and she goes to Poly Cocktails. But most people who go just use it to find other poly people so that they can have off-site . . . parties."

"Sex parties!?" I say, still too loud. I'm thankful for the noise of crying toddlers.

"No, Molly," says Stew. "Tupperware parties. What do you think? Can I finish this story, please?"

"Right. Sorry."

"So the parties are kind of curated—no more than four or five couples, and everyone has to get an STD test beforehand. Tinkerbell was hosting, and she asked me to be her date. So I went." The waitress comes back with Stew's card. He thanks her and starts to sign. "Let's go," he says to me.

"Wait, you can't leave the story there!"

"I'll tell you while we walk. The play's about to start."

As we walk, Stewart fills in a few details. When he got to the party, he felt self-conscious—everyone there was under forty. He and Tinkerbell fooled around, but he didn't feel particularly attracted to her. This was only their second meeting, and he hadn't seen her naked before.

"She has tattoos all over her back, and her nipples are pierced," he says. "You know I'm not into that stuff."

"Uh-huh," I say, feeling gratitude to Stewart for relating only the negatives of the experience—which is to say, the details I can handle. But like a fool, I push for more. "Was there anything you liked about it?"

"Of course," says Stew, too quickly. And then, before I can retract my question, he adds, "It's like having a front-row seat for porn. It was kinda cool watching other people get off, you know?"

I nod, mute, tears rising. I blink them away. We're at Nate's school now, and I look forward to an hour in a dark auditorium to process what Stewart has just told me. Nate is playing a newspaper salesman and is in only one scene—toward the end, he says—so I've got some time in which to zone out.

The feeling behind the tears is a familiar one. It is my worry, my fear, that I don't fulfill all of Stewart's needs. He likes to watch people having sex. And—not for lack of trying—I can't give that to him.

But a new thought is dawning on me while I watch, as if from a great distance, children tripping across the stage and forgetting lines, parents in the rows ahead of me angling phones for the perfect shot of their little stars.

What does it matter if Stew gets some of his needs met elsewhere? I think. And behind this thought is a new feeling, too—a tingling of freedom. If I'm no longer Stew's only sex partner, then there's no guilt in saying no to things I don't want to do. This is a good thing, right? Win-win! So why do I still feel jealous? Why is this feeling of compersion so elusive?

"Extra! Extra! Read all about it!" I hear Nate's voice booming behind me. Every head in the auditorium turns in the direction of the sound. I fumble for my phone and see with relief that Stew is already videotaping. There is our little boy, strutting down the aisle, adorable and confident. It is without a doubt Nate's scene. A showstopper. He gets more laughs than anyone, and takes a dramatic bow before exiting stage left.

Stewart stops the video and grabs my hand, kisses it, and continues to hold it tight. He leans over and whispers in my ear, "I love you." And I realize that our marriage is safe. Never mind that I won't go to a sex party with him. There is nothing that could bond me to Stewart more than our common love objects: our children.

———

ON SUNDAY, I GET another text from Liam: *Really hoping u can make it to Poly Cocktails tomorrow. 2 of my partners coming— would love for you to meet them. LMK!*

I race back to *The Ethical Slut* and pore through the index, looking for help. I ricochet between sections titled "A Slut Utopia," "Circles and Tribes," and "Relationship Boundaries." Within a span of ten minutes, I convince myself I'd love nothing more than to hang out with Liam's stunning girlfriends, irrationally worry that Tinkerbell will be among them, and finally decide to skip the whole thing. Although *The Ethical Slut* assures me at every step that I should be gentle with myself, that I should feel comfortable saying no and doing what's right for me, I feel neurotic and unevolved.

I don't think that scene is for me, I write to Liam. *But thanks so much for the invite. I've learned a lot from you!*

I hit Send and breathe a sigh of relief, the door to this branch of the "poly community" safely shut behind me.

TO KEEP MY MIND off the quadruple date I'm not going on, I spend Monday night scouring OkCupid. Maybe what I need isn't a poly professor but an open-relationship rookie, someone who has as many questions as I do about this entire world. As I read through the dozens of messages in my inbox, one of them catches my eye. A close-up picture of a boyish, bearded, smiling face accompanies the profile:

Name: Karl
Age: 36
Height: 6'3"
Body Type: A little extra
Relationship Status: Ethically Non-monogamous (partnered)

Hallo, writes Karl. *You seem very interesting. You are a teacher? Maybe you can help me with my Grammar! I am German and I love the Grammar Girl podcast! (2nd place to The Moth.) We can trade lessons: Backgammon for Grammar!*

His enthusiasm is refreshing: no games—other than backgammon, of course. I silently praise my OKC Premium account for letting me know that he's currently online. I type quickly.

Hi there, Karl. That sounds like fun. Where do you live?

Ah, you are in the cyberspace now too! I am living in Windsor Terrace. You?

I hesitate. Windsor Terrace is awfully close. But Stewart will be so thrilled I've found someone I like, I'm sure he'll overlook the "no one in the neighborhood" rule.

I'm in Park Slope! I write back. *May I ask you about your ENM status? Are you married? Have you been in an open relationship for long?*

Not married yet. I and my fiancée, Martina, live together. We have been open for about 6 months. You?

Married 16 years, I reply. *Open for a while but still figuring it out. And here's your first grammar lesson: "My fiancée and I"—personal pronoun comes second.*

Wow. Personal pronoun?! This is like foreplay for me! LOL.

I can't stand *LOL,* but since I *am* laughing out loud, I decide to let it pass. *Then we'll get along just fine,* I write.

KARL AND I SET a date for Thursday night, at Lucey's Lounge on Third Avenue—in the direction of Gowanus, where neighbors and mothers of my kids' friends won't be likely to tread. It's less than a ten-minute walk, but I leave a half hour early and take a circuitous route. I need time to think.

Karl and I have already exchanged dozens of texts over the previous three days. He asks me lots of questions about English grammar—finer points, such as when to use the subjunctive and the difference between *less* and *fewer*—which earns my respect. He tells me about his work as a freelance photographer and asks me about my life. On Wednesday he sends me a voice memo so I can hear his accent—"Hallo, Molly. This is Karl. Now you are sure I am very German!" His voice is friendly—and the quirks of his inflected English beyond charming.

Most importantly, I learn from Karl that he and his fiancée, Martina, have been discussing the possibility of an open relationship for years. The arrangement was even her idea. Martina is bisexual and wants female intimacy in her life. Karl tells me they're learning a lot—together—and it's going well. I feel a certain degree of safety in the parallel nature of our experiences. Maybe this will be a relationship that can last. Maybe Karl will be the person who can fill up my empty places. Maybe we'll fall in . . .

The glimmer of this thought simultaneously makes me giddy with anticipation and heavies my legs with a leaden dread. *No falling in love* still tops our list of relationship statutes. But is this a rule I want to follow? Have I already broken it? I'm still not sure how to classify the feelings I had for Matt, but I know I did have feelings. I also know that my relationships with Leo and Laurent were primarily about sex—and they left me cold.

The Ethical Slut has taken up permanent residency in my nightstand drawer, and I turn to it again and again, looking for answers. The chapter called "Making Agreements" is now filled with dog-eared pages and highlighted passages. I fixate on one paragraph in particular:

> *Janet and one of her partners, for example, began their*
> *relationship with an agreement that they could be sexual with*

other people, but that they couldn't fall in love with anyone else.
Then one of them did. (In hindsight, this seems like a fairly silly
agreement—as though you could simply decide not to fall in
love!)

These words offer equal parts terror and comfort. Is our no-falling-in-love agreement destined to change? And could I actually love somebody else without threatening my marriage?

I shove these thoughts into a quivering corner of my mind and turn my attention to the last block separating me from my first date with Karl. As I approach the bar, I see a large figure in a dark coat standing in the middle of the sidewalk, furiously blowing his nose into what appears to be a real live handkerchief. He looks up and sees me walking toward him. His face lights up in a huge smile, even as he's still vigorously wiping his nose with his hankie. It's Karl. The man is already showing me his boogers. There is something about the vulnerability of this act—the complete lack of pretense—that sends a dizzying wave from my heart to my pelvis and back again.

Karl tucks his handkerchief into his pocket and opens his arms. He is quite literally as large as a bear, and he crushes me in a strong embrace. His woolen coat is infused with the smell of cigarettes. And although I've never dated a smoker, I am instantly drawn to the aroma. He seems so nice, so proper—but the smoke is proof of a destructive streak, giving him a bad-boy edge. After a moment, Karl releases me.

"So you are Molly?" he asks, looking into my face, still beaming.

"You probably should have asked that before you hugged me."

He laughs. Fully. Easily. "This is true. Shall we go inside?"

"I'd love to."

LATER THAT NIGHT, I'M in bed with Stew. He's asked about my date with Karl, and I'm finding it difficult to tell him anything without tipping my hand. If I tell him the smallest part of the truth—that I had a great time—I'll prove Stewart's point: that my interest in keeping our marriage open is dependent on who I'm dating at the moment. Then what happens if my relationship with Karl goes south and I want to close the marriage after all? What leg will I have to stand on when Stewart assures me that I'll change my mind as soon as I meet someone new?

And then, if I go deeper into the truth—if I reveal that I'm *feeling* things for another person—I'm not sure what will happen. Will Stew shrug it off, not believing I could be so enraptured after a single date? Will he be angry and hurt and accuse me of crossing a line? Or will it be worse than that? Will he confess that he, too, has developed feelings for someone else?

To avoid these imaginary scenarios, I give incomplete answers to his questions.

"What did you guys talk about?" he asks.

"You know. Usual first-date stuff. Jobs. Families," I say. I don't say that Karl showed me some of his photographs, that they are evidence of a beautiful soul. I don't say that Karl told me about the death of his father, that he started to tear up as he did so. And that I did, too.

"Okay," says Stew, eyeing me suspiciously. When it comes to most topics, he can't get me to shut up. "So what does he look like? No, wait. Let me guess. I'll bet he's another Anti-Stew—tall, skinny, and a full head of hair."

"He's definitely tall," I answer, "but he's far from skinny. And his hair is thinning a bit on top. See?" I show him the profile picture on OkCupid, relishing the surprise on his face as he takes in Karl's girth, glasses, and regular-guy looks. This is exactly how I need Stewart to feel: unthreatened.

"Did you kiss him?"

My mind swoons at the memory of our first kiss. We were sitting on the couch in the bar's back room, and as soon as the only other patrons left, Karl leaned toward me, a hand on my knee, and said in his staccato English, "I really want to kiss you. Would that be all right?"

I nodded and he kissed me. The most tender first kiss I've ever experienced, sensual rather than sexual, his bushy beard so much softer than I'd expected, his thick fingers brushing my cheek.

"Yup," I say to Stew.

"And?"

"It was nice."

"Just nice?" He emphasizes the question with his eyes.

"Yeah," I say. "It was just nice."

Just nice is exactly what I crave.

CHAPTER 11

"I HAVE SOME NEWS," my mother tells me over the phone as I sit on my bed folding laundry.

"Yeah?" I ask distractedly. My mother's news usually has to do with which flowers are blooming in the yard or updates on the lives of people from my childhood whom I barely remember. I've got more pressing matters on my mind: Karl. I'm seeing him again tonight—three times in one week. For our second date, we went out to dinner and then to a Moth StorySLAM at the Bell House. We got there too late to snag seats, so Karl stood behind me as we watched the storytellers, his hands resting on my hips, inviting me to lean back onto his sturdy frame and inhale his smoky skin. Unlike Laurent's groping, Karl's touch feels easeful, as if my hips are his final destination. And tonight, while his fiancée is out with her girlfriend, Karl has invited me over to their apartment.

This afternoon, while Daniel and Nate turned the living room into a cushion fort, I'd read the section of *The Ethical Slut* on something called new relationship energy, or NRE. I think Karl has given me a full-blown case. Straight-A Molly has even highlighted the relevant passages and nearly committed them to memory:

> *Many people new to open relationships try to limit outside sexual encounters to a casual, recreational level to avoid the terrifying specter of seeing your partner in love with, or at least crushed out*

*on, another. . . . We certainly do not want to draw the boundaries
of our agreements so tightly that we exclude everybody we like.
There is no rule that will protect us from our own emotions.*

The Ethical Slut went on to remind me that new relationships
are exciting because they *are* new. That the honeymoon phase of
every relationship ends. That a new relationship needn't threaten
the deeper intimacy I have with my husband. But it doesn't tell me
what to *do* with this energy coursing through my body—a frenetic
vibration in the same frequency as what I felt with Matt. There
is something reassuring, though, about the fact that I've felt this
before. If our marriage survived Matt, it can survive Karl, right?
But what about me? Can *I* survive another tsunami of the heart?
Even now, multitasking on my bed, talking to my mother while
folding laundry, I can't get him out of my mind.

"I went to see a new doctor yesterday," my mother continues.

"Uh-huh . . ." Doctor visits are another frequent topic. The list
of neurological disorders my mother does *not* have seems to grow
with every appointment. She doesn't have an excess of heavy metals
in her blood. She doesn't have chronic Lyme disease. She doesn't
have a brain tumor, or MS, or an inner ear infection. Yet her body
continues to slow down in every conceivable way. Walking, getting
up from the toilet, even lifting a fork to her mouth—it's all more
difficult with each passing day.

"A new neurologist," she says. "She's quite sure I have a form
of Parkinson's disease."

I freeze, a pair of Stewart's boxers suspended mid-fold in front
of me.

"What?" Leave it to my mother to declare this diagnosis in
the same tone she'd use to announce the graduation of a former
colleague's grandson. "I thought the Mayo Clinic ruled out Parkinson's years ago."

"This doctor seems to think they were wrong. She called it Park-in-son-is-m. Whoo! That's hard to say."

"So what does this mean?"

"I'm not sure," my mother answers slowly. "But it could be very good news. She's starting me on a medication called Sinemet. If it works, I could be moving a lot better within a couple of weeks."

"What? Mom, that's amazing! So have you already started on this drug?" I hold my breath, thinking about her past aversion to Western medicine. She held so tightly to Mahikari's belief that all illness was toxins moving out of the body. I hope she's past those ideas by now.

"Yes," she says. I exhale.

"Have you noticed any changes?"

"Well, it's hard to say. But I think I do! I feel like I have a bit more energy. But maybe . . ." Her voice cracks with emotion. "Maybe it's just the return of hope."

A mishmash of feelings rises within me, too. "This is wonderful news, Mom. You've been through so much. You deserve some hope."

"Oh, sweetheart," she says. "Thank you."

THAT NIGHT, I WALK to Karl's apartment at the edge of Green-Wood Cemetery. As I make my way along the last block, hemmed in on one side by silent graves, I stop to check my face in the side-view mirror of a parked car. I want to give my reflection some words of encouragement, but thoughts are slow to form. They remain jumbled as I walk up the stoop and ring the second bell, labeled with both Karl's and Martina's names. I see Karl emerge at the end of the hallway, taking long strides toward me as he breaks into a grin. I smile back.

He opens the door and kisses me on the lips.

I look warily at the door marked #1, immediately to our right, and Karl waves a hand. "Not to worry. The neighbors are our friends. They know all about Martina and me."

He takes me by the hand and leads me through door #2. I feel like a character in a Choose Your Own Adventure book. As I enter the apartment, I know I've chosen well. I find myself in an adult, feminine-inflected wonderland, a home that is neither overrun by children nor a bachelor's pad. A few candles are lit, and a bouquet of flowers is on the small kitchen table. Acoustic guitar music plays on the stereo, and a bottle of wine and two glasses have been laid out on the counter.

Karl gathers me into his arms and kisses me again, deeply this time. "I have looked forward to having you here since your very first text," he says. "But where are my manners? Please, let me take your coat. Take off your shoes, too, if you like. It's nice and cozy in here." As he hangs up my coat and starts to pour the wine, I walk into the living room, my feet sinking into a deep shag rug that's free of cookie crumbs and hidden Legos. The walls are covered with framed photographs, some of which I recognize from the work Karl showed me on his phone on our first date.

"Make yourself comfortable," Karl says, handing me a glass of wine. I lean back onto the couch cushions, and he pats his lap. "Give me your feet. I give very good massages."

"Are you kidding?" I say, looking around the apartment for a hidden camera.

"Why would this be a joke?" Karl asks, smiling as he peels off my socks and begins to knead one instep with a strong thumb. It takes all my effort not to moan aloud.

"Not a joke," I say. "It's just—your apartment has a very different vibe than my house. I feel like I've walked into a spa."

He laughs. "This is why I'm a homebody." He raises my foot into the air and kisses me delicately on one toe. I'm thankful I squeezed in a pedicure yesterday. "And I am very happy to have you in our home."

The word *our* jolts me for a moment, but my mind is quick to smooth over any discomfort. *This is what it's all about,* I tell myself, taking another sip of wine. I'm dating a man who's in the same situation I am. We both have partners whom we live with, whom we love. And the perks of this arrangement are starting to become apparent. Karl clearly knows how to keep a woman happy.

I put my wineglass down and close my eyes. Karl's hands are working their way up my calves now. And then he is touching my thighs, peeling off my leggings and pressing the heel of his hand against the front of my panties. I feel his breath on my face and keep my eyes shut as he kisses me and moves his fingers gently along the seam of my pussy, never quite parting the lips. I have never been touched this softly, this gently. It's the sweetest agony I've ever experienced. I'm writhing on the couch when Karl stops.

"May I undress you?"

"Yes."

He takes my hands and pulls me to my feet. I stand, an ache between my legs as he lifts my dress over my head and folds it neatly on the end table. He smiles at the front clasp of my bra and unhooks it, pausing to kiss me on each nipple before placing the bra carefully on top of the dress. He gets down on his knees and slowly removes my panties. My legs shake as he kisses me gently just below my belly button.

"Come with me," he says, standing back up.

In the bedroom, I lie down on hotel-grade sheets. The lights are dimmed, and a candle glows on the bedside table. The same acoustic guitar comes through hidden speakers, so that the space is infused with music. The plucks and strums are connected to Karl's light touch. He is sounding my body like a precious instrument, searching for previously unheard notes. His fingers and his mouth move fluidly, fusing with my skin. I am something new, something so glorious that when I finally orgasm, I have no words. I feel like an exploding star, awash in light and colors that can be expressed only through music and sensation. The sound of my own scream and the wet tears on my face bring me back to myself. Karl's smiling face hovers above me, and I grab for him, weeping into his neck.

"That was enjoyable for you?" he asks, and I laugh through my sobs.

"I don't even know what that was!" I say when I find my voice. It's then that I notice Karl is still completely dressed. "But what about you?"

He kisses me on the nose. "Don't worry about me. I get pleasure from giving *you* pleasure."

"Really?" I say. "How did I get so lucky?"

"I am the lucky one. You relax. I will be right back."

He leaves me lying on the bed and disappears into the living room. The music still fills the air, scented by the lavender candle, and I stare at the ceiling, sighing contentedly, my mind devoid of thought. I roll onto my side and notice for the first time a huge black-and-white photograph looming above me. It's a woman's naked body, lying facedown on a bed. I sit up and stare at her narrow waist, her perfectly formed buttocks, the body of a master craftsman's cello. Her cheek is turned to the side, but a mass of blond curly hair blocks her face. I look more closely and notice that the headboard in the photo matches the one I now lean against, where identical pillows are arranged.

Karl returns with our wineglasses, refilled.

"Who is that?" I say, hoping my voice sounds neutral.

"That," says Karl, smiling broadly, "is Martina. Isn't she beautiful?"

LATER, KARL VOLUNTEERS TO walk me to 10th Street, but I put him off, saying he should be home to greet Martina when she returns. I need to think, to use the mile separating his apartment from my house—such a laughably short distance, considering the gulf between decadence and responsibility it represents—to make sense of what I'm feeling.

I've clung to my role as Stewart's "primary" partner, his wife, the mother of his children. When Stew goes out with other women, he comes home to *me,* always assuring me that I'm the only one he will ever want to make a life with. And though I've chosen Karl largely because he is in a similar relationship with Martina, albeit without the children and years of marriage, I've never thought about what it means to be the "secondary" partner—until now.

The woman in the photograph is the woman Karl considers the pinnacle of beauty, the woman he wants to be with forever, the woman he loves. This rouses in me feelings of jealousy I thought were reserved only for Stewart. But Martina is also the woman who created the sanctuary I just enjoyed, who chose the scented candles and high-thread-count sheets, who stayed away from *her* home so that I could be tenderly ministered to by *her* man. And for this, I am deeply grateful. I feel intrigued—drawn and connected to her—in a way that surprises me.

As I climb the steps of our stoop, I feel my phone buzz in my pocket. I pull it out and see a text from Karl.

I hope you have gotten home safely! he's written.

I smile. Is it possible that Karl is the first man (other than Stewart, of course) to worry about my well-being after a date? I'm filled with a pleasant fluttering. *Yes, I'm at my front door now,* I write back. *Thank you for a wonderful evening.*

It was wonderful for me, too, he says. I see three dots forming into another text, and I wait with my key in the lock, not wanting to enter my Lego-strewn living room and break Karl's spell just yet. The next message arrives:

Martina is glad I didn't change the sheets after you left. She likes the smell of you.

I stare at the message. With my eyes still on my phone, I turn the key and walk through the door. I jump when I see Stewart standing in front of me.

"Nice to see you too, baby," he says, leaning forward to kiss me.

"Sorry, I wasn't expecting you to be home. Didn't you have a date tonight?"

A couple of weeks ago, after Nate turned eleven, the boys argued that they no longer needed a babysitter. After all, Daniel was almost fourteen. Stew and I went out for a local dinner as a test run, and when we returned home at ten o'clock, Daniel announced that Nate was in bed—something I rarely achieved so early.

"How did you do it?" I asked.

"I let him play video games with me, and then I set a timer to see how fast he could brush his teeth and put on his pajamas. And I told him if he wasn't in bed before you guys got home, we'd never get to stay by ourselves again," he said smugly. I had to admit that not needing a babysitter was a life-changing development. Especially when both boys seemed genuinely excited to stay home alone together.

"Yup," Stewart says as I take off my coat and boots. "But guess what? I went out with a woman who's also in an open marriage. With three kids, too. And she had to get home by midnight. She lives in New Jersey."

"Wow," I say. Recently, Stewart has dated a string of single women. He ended things with the last one when she asked if he would ever divorce me. He told her there was no chance of that, and she broke into tears.

"I thought you'd like that," he says.

"I do." A woman with her own life, her own husband, her own kids? A woman who doesn't want more than Stewart is able to give? "That's really great."

"So how was your date with Karl?" he asks, his voice lowering suggestively.

I know he wants to hear about the sex, but that's not what I want to talk about. For one, it feels too special, too precious. I don't want to cheapen it by describing it in terms that will turn Stewart on. Besides, the Martina situation is what I truly need to discuss.

"It was fun," I say, sitting down on the couch, "but I'm not sure how to handle something." I tell him about the naked photograph of Martina, her comment about my smell on the sheets.

"Interesting," he says, the growl still in his voice. "So you came all over the sheets, huh? Tell me more." He takes my feet onto his lap and starts to rub. I can't remember the last time I got a foot massage, let alone two in one night.

"That's not the point," I say. "Don't you think that's a little weird? It makes me—I don't know—uncomfortable."

"Baby," he says, his tone returning to normal. "I think it's a good thing. That means she's actually into you coming over. You said it was fun, right?"

"Yeah."

"And you already knew she's bisexual. She was at her girl-friend's place tonight?"

"Yeah," I say again. "That part's a little weird, too. Her girlfriend—I think her name is Rebecca—is also engaged. To a man. And Karl told me Martina is the first woman Rebecca ever slept with. He says Martina likes 'straight chicks.'"

Stew laughs. "Well, they must not be *that* straight if they're having sex with her."

"Exactly," I say. "Don't you think that's weird?"

"Not at all," says Stew. "Granted, I'm not a bisexual woman. But it's a pretty popular male fantasy to get a lesbian to 'turn straight.' Maybe she's into the same sort of thing, but in reverse. That's her kink."

"Maybe," I say, still feeling doubts I can't put my finger on.

"Think of it this way," he says, still rubbing my feet. "Look how much we're learning about other people. It's like we have this intimate window into the lives of people we might otherwise never even meet. I think it's kind of cool."

"It is pretty crazy how much I already know about Martina. And how much she probably knows about me."

Stew laughs. "Kiwi already thinks you're amazing, too. But that's because I only tell her the good stuff." He winks at me.

"Kiwi?"

"The woman I went out with tonight—the one from New Jersey, who's in an open marriage. She's originally from New Zealand. So that's my nickname for her."

A knot starts to twist in my stomach. A nickname? Stewart has a million nicknames for me—Vasco da Gama when I get lost, Mario Andretti when I get a speeding ticket, the ever-favored Suitcase. But a nickname for another woman? And one that conjures up an unbearably cute accent? I try to shove my jealousy to the side and probe the other part of what Stewart said, the part that should make me feel *good*.

"What did you tell her about me?"

"That you're beautiful. And funny. That you're an amazing mother, and wife, and friend, and daughter."

Daughter. A wave of guilt washes over me. "Oh my God," I say. "I can't believe I forgot to tell you. I talked to my mom today. She found a new doctor who might be able to help her."

———

THAT NIGHT, AS I spoon into Stewart, I feel like I've taken a handful of uppers and downers in one careless gulp. On the one hand, everything is perfect. I feel connected to Stewart. And although jealousy is still my frequent companion, I'm starting to observe it for what it is: a feeling that is sometimes unwarranted. Stew may have a cute nickname for his new girlfriend (*should I even use the g-word?*), but he also tells her about me, about how much he loves me. And she has a husband and children of her own. Not a threat at all, right? Then there's Karl. I've found a man who is sweet and attentive and clearly into me who also has his own primary relationship. This is sustainable, right? On top of that, my kids are becoming more independent. They're starting to stay home alone—and are enjoying it. And like a cherry on top of the sundae, my mom has hope for her health for the first time in more than a decade. So what is it that's making me so anxious? Why can't I trust that everything is okay? I pull Stewart's arm closer to me and hang on tight, falling into a fitful sleep.

THE NEXT DAY, I decide to give myself a break and head back to the shallows of OkCupid. A quick fling might cure me of my growing attachment to Karl, and distract me from obsessing over Stewart's dating life and my mother's health. I just need some light-hearted fun.

I decide to reach out to a guy I've been out with once—just for drinks—who's also in an open relationship. Besides being cute and sweet, Jay would help me set a personal record. He's fourteen years younger than I am. I hardly stop to consider whether this is an attempt to level the playing field with Stewart—he let slip that Kiwi is thirteen years his junior (and thus eight years younger than I am). But Stew claims her being married with three kids, not to mention making a life for herself in a new country, balances this out.

"She's lived more than an average thirty-five-year-old. And anyway, it's half plus seven, right?" he says, referring to our agreed-upon formula for determining if a potential partner is too young. According to this rule, Stewart, at forty-eight, is allowed to date thirty-one-year-olds. At forty-three, I can dip down to twenty-eight and a half. Jay is a ripe old twenty-nine. And although he was heading out of town for a few weeks after that first date, I now see that I have an unread message from him in my inbox.

Hey Molly, it says. *I'm back from my wilderness adventure and would love to see you again. Let me know when you have a free evening!* He signs off with his phone number.

I smile at the memory of Jay telling me he was going camping with his girlfriend. *This is why non-monogamy is great,* I think. *I will never, ever sleep in a tent with Jay. But he can camp to his heart's content with somebody else!*

Since he's sent me his number, I ditch the app and text him.

Hi, Jay! It's Molly. So glad you're back. What are you up to tomorrow night?

I AGREE TO GO to Jay's apartment this time. His girlfriend will be spending the night with her *other* boyfriend to accommodate us. Jay lives in Queens, and I have to take two trains to get there. Just before I leave, I receive a text from Karl.

Hallo, Molly. What are you up to this evening?

I hesitate for a moment but decide to tell the truth.

Hi, Karl, I write. *I'm going on a second date with someone. Unfortunately, he lives in Queens.* I punctuate this with a frowning emoji, hoping to make Karl feel that this date is more a bother than a pleasure. *I'm still seeing you on Friday, yes?* To this I add the emoji with the clapping hands.

The three dots hover for a moment, and then I see his reply: *Oh yes. I am looking forward to Friday! Have fun tonight!*

I feel relief at his response, and smugness at the beauty of my life. I can have two cakes *and* a husband, too. But by the time I've disembarked from the N train and walked an additional twelve blocks in freezing rain, I'm rethinking the benefits of seeing anyone other than Karl.

Jay buzzes me in through the front door of a nondescript highrise, and I search for the elevator bank that will take me to his floor. My shoes and umbrella are dripping, and I'm sure my hair and makeup look nothing like they did when I left my house more than an hour ago. I try to coax a small spark of nerves into a larger blaze of desire, but my body is too cold and soggy to burn.

I walk through the mazelike corridors on the eighth floor, looking for apartment 8N.

The walls are marred by gray smudges and chipped paint, and I'm starting to feel claustrophobic. I've reached an emergency exit and have turned back toward the elevators when I see a door open at the end of the hallway. Jay pops his head out. In the harsh fluorescent lighting, he looks much younger than I remember. There is a trace of stubble on his jawline, but I doubt he could grow a full beard. His oxford shirt is tucked into belted jeans, making him look like a geeky teenager on Picture Day.

"Hi, Molly," he says, waving. "Sorry, this building is kind of confusing."

"Hi," I reply, smoothing down my hair. I put my umbrella on his front mat and we hug awkwardly. "Oh no. I'm getting you wet."

"Don't worry about it," he says. "You can just drop your coat over here."

Drop is exactly what he means. There really isn't a place to hang a coat, so I leave mine in an unceremonious puddle. I follow him into a vast, couch-less living room. A TV takes up one entire wall, and a couple of cushions are on the floor.

"Wow," I say, trying to sound positive. "This place is really spacious. How long have you lived here?" I want to give him the benefit of the doubt. Maybe they just moved in?

"Um, like a year and a half?" he says. And then, as if he's read my thoughts but not the full subtext, he adds, "Our couch broke—it was a secondhand IKEA piece of shit—and we never bothered to replace it."

"Got it."

"Do you want to see the bedroom?" he asks, sounding nervous.

"Sure," I say. After all, that's what I'm here for, right?

The bedroom, thankfully, is fully furnished. The bed is even made—with new sheets, I hope, though I try not to overthink it. The lights are on full blast, and the predominant sound is the traffic humming along the Brooklyn-Queens Expressway. I wonder if Jay is going to do something about the atmosphere. I don't need candles and music, necessarily, but a dimmer switch might be nice.

Instead, Jay grabs me by the waist and pulls me toward him, kissing me with closed lips just once and reading my face for permission before jamming his tongue into my mouth.

"I want to eat your pussy," he says, using the same tone of voice with which he told me about the broken couch.

"Okay," I say. I've worn an outfit that's easy on, easy off. With a few deft movements, I'm naked, lying on the bed, and watching Jay as he wrestles with his belt, the buttons of his shirt, his jeans, his socks. I notice with surprise that bulging inside his boxer briefs is the biggest cock I've ever seen. The promise of his package serves to make me instantaneously wet.

Before I can even settle myself against the pillows, Jay pounces on my pussy like a dog with a chew toy, more teeth than tongue. I put my hands on his head, but he doesn't take the cue. I wait what feels like a polite interval, then divert him with a tactful compliment rather than a criticism.

"Why don't you fuck me with that big cock of yours instead? Do you have a condom? I brought some just in case, but they're—um—regular-sized."

Jay smiles sheepishly. "Just a second." He turns to the dresser and takes a box from the top drawer.

"Wow. I didn't even know Magnum XL was a thing!"

"Yeah," he says, laughing. "I've had to shop around a bit."

"I can only imagine." I watch in awe as he kicks off his underwear and unrolls the condom along his considerable length and girth.

"You ready?"

"Definitely."

Jay gets on top of me and guides his massive, rubber-encased dick inside me. I close my eyes and wait to feel something new. But this is a familiar sensation, and not a good one. As Jay earnestly thrusts, I feel like I'm in the gynecologist's chair and a speculum is being slammed against my cervix. I raise my hips and try moving them in a circle. Surely some part of this massive cock will touch my G-spot if I maneuver correctly, right? But no dice.

Although it isn't painful, it certainly isn't pleasant. And yet, I catch myself making sounds of enjoyment. *Speak up, Molly,* I say to myself. *Have you truly learned nothing?*

"Mmm . . ." I fake-moan. "I want you to take me from behind."

"Okay," says Jay. He backs off of me, and I crawl to the edge of the bed, avoiding eye contact. Doggie-style, his cock feels less like a medical instrument and more like a rigid dildo, the kind I used once or twice in my twenties and then discarded, realizing that nothing beats actual flesh and blood. The advantage now is that I can touch my own clit, and within a minute or two, as I ignore the slamming behind me, I conjure a tingle and decide to call it an orgasm. I moan a little louder and shake my hips.

"Are you done?" he asks me.

"Yeah," I lie. "That was great. Do you want to come, too?" I hope he's close.

He pulls out of me and takes off his condom. "I usually can't come through intercourse," he says apologetically. A pang of sympathy washes over me. *Poor kid,* I think before I can stop myself.

"How do you usually come then?" I ask. I'm praying he doesn't ask for a blow job. The thought of trying to fit him into my mouth is horrifying. All these years, I've been led to believe that big cocks are the best thing since sliced bread. I suddenly feel immense gratitude for the perfection of Stewart's penis, for the various ways he brings me to orgasm. And then I think of Karl, his sincerity in telling me he gets pleasure from *my* pleasure. What am I even doing here?

"To be honest," Jay answers, "masturbation is my go-to." I internally sigh with relief. "But don't get me wrong. You're super sexy. And I'm totally going to think about you when I get myself off later."

"You're sweet," I say. And I mean it, albeit in a way that feels almost maternal. He may be almost thirty, but I feel like Jay and I are in different generations. Probably because we are.

On my way to the subway, I pull out my phone to text Stewart—*Heading home and thanking the heavens for your perfectly sized penis!*—and see there are three messages from Karl.

The first one puts a smile on my face: *Molly, I hope you are having a nice date.*

The second one erases it: *That was a lie. I hope the date is terrible. I'm feeling very jealous although I have no right to be.*

The third one makes my heart ache for Karl and my appreciation for Martina grow: *Martina thinks I should stop texting and let you have your freedom, but I can't help myself. I don't know what is wrong with me. I'm sorry.*

The last message was sent just minutes earlier, so I call him instead of writing back.

"Molly?" he answers on the first ring. "Please forgive all the texts. I am a mess."

"It's okay, Karl," I say. "I wanted to tell you how awful my date was! I'm already on my way home."

"Really? You're not trying to make me feel better?" And then, hurriedly: "Because you're allowed to have a nice date."

I laugh. "No, he's a decent guy, but I have no interest in seeing him again. Honestly." I decide not to tell Karl the anatomical reason for this decision and again feel a wave of gratitude for Stewart. Stew could never tell me that a woman's gigantic breasts were problematic during sex, but I know I can tell *him* anything. We'll have a good laugh together over the Case of the Enormous Schlong.

Karl exhales deeply. "I'm so glad, but I shouldn't behave like this. I don't know what got into me! Can you forgive me?"

"Of course," I say. Rather than being annoyed, I'm flattered. "There's nothing to forgive. You just told me how you're feeling."

"Yes," he says. "But this is not something we talked about before. I know you are free to date whomever you like." I silently give him points for using *whomever* correctly—a grammar topic from our early texts. "But for myself, I am disabling my OkCupid account. I would only like to date you. Would that be all right?"

I think about the hour-plus subway ride to Jay's apartment, the barren living room, the ridiculously bad sex. Why did I even have this date? What am I trying to prove?

"Actually, Karl," I say, and my heart fills in a way that is both lovely and terrifying, "I'd like the same thing. I'll disable my account tonight, too."

"You will?" he says, unable to contain the excitement in his voice. "I am not pressuring you?"

"Not at all. Tonight's date was *that* bad." He laughs, and I allow myself to add, "And you are *that* wonderful." I mean it. I truly have no interest in seeing anyone else.

"Molly, it is *you* who are wonderful," he says. My legs melt under me and I stop walking to enjoy the sensation. "I am so relieved we talked. I thought I might die of jealousy tonight. Martina tried to help, but I pouted all evening. It was very bad."

"But this can't be the first time you've felt this way," I say. "Don't you get jealous when Martina is out with somebody else?"

"With Martina, it's easy," he responds. "She only dates women, and I *like* to imagine two women together." He falls into a whisper. "For example, if I knew that you were out with Martina, I would not be jealous at all."

I manage a weak laugh. Surely he's joking. "I'll see you on Friday?"

"I cannot wait."

I GO TO KARL'S apartment on Friday. And on Sunday afternoon. And again on Tuesday evening. He introduces me to new wine (*I think you would like a nice tart Grüner*), new music (*You don't know First Aid Kit? They are from Sweden. Very special*), and new ways of being during sex.

Karl is a gentle lover—a change from the dominance of Leo, Laurent, and Stewart. I've always believed I needed a man who is in control. With Stew, I barely have to think, and most of the time, I enjoy the submissive role. Stewart especially knows how I like to be held down—never to the point of pain, but with enough pressure that I can orgasm fully, can empty myself out again and again and again. Stew has explained to me more than once that to stay hard for an hour, sometimes longer, he must conjure the self-restraint of a machine. This sometimes leads to the vocal expulsion of pent-up energy, often in the form of words like *cunt* and *whore*.

"I swear I'm not doing it on purpose. It just kind of comes out." When I complain, it takes him out of the moment. Over time, we've arrived at a compromise, less than satisfactory for both of us: He will try his best not to scream *cunt* during sex, and I will do my best to ignore him if he does.

But I never realized that what I crave isn't the absence of vulgarities but the presence of something else. So when Karl whispers in my ear, "What do you want?," I surprise myself with the immediacy of my answer.

"I want you to call me a good girl," I say.

After that, sex with Karl becomes a kind of affirmation, body and soul. "You're such a good girl, Molly," he coos in bed in his cute German accent. He makes me orgasm with his mouth, his fingers, his cock, and combinations thereof. I almost always cry when Karl makes me come. Sometimes he cries, too.

A FEW WEEKS LATER, at couples therapy, Evelyn asks an open-ended question: "So how are things going with you two?"

"Things are great," I say. "I think we're both really happy."

"I'm glad to hear that," says Evelyn. "Why do you think that is?"

"Well, we're each dating someone now, and it's going well, so I think that helps." I glance over at Stewart and am surprised to see that he's staring at his hands in his lap. "Don't you agree?"

"I guess so," says Stew. "But it's more like *I'm* doing pretty well, and *you're* doing pretty well. But I don't feel like *we* are doing well."

"That's crazy!" I say.

"Molly," Evelyn says gently. "Remember, feelings aren't facts.

Let Stewart finish. How would you characterize your relationship with Molly lately?"

"It's hard to say, exactly," says Stew. "This guy she's dating, Karl. He lives nearby, and I feel like she's always running over to his apartment. And when she's not over there, she's texting him or talking about him. I know she's excited to have found someone she likes. But I feel like she's not really present with me anymore. Like what happened the other night."

His voice breaks, and he looks back at his hands. I stare at him, dumbfounded. I rack my brain, trying to think of what he might be talking about. Evelyn notices.

"Stewart, could you tell Molly what happened that made you feel like she wasn't present?"

He exhales and grips his thighs, as if willing his fingers not to ball into fists. "Do you remember on Sunday? When you were making dinner, and the kids were playing video games, and I was working in the dining room?"

I nod, still confused.

"I remember thinking how nice it was that we were all home. And then I came into the kitchen to get something to drink, and I saw your phone. I wasn't trying to invade your privacy, I just glanced over. I saw your text to Karl."

I look at Stewart's face, but his eyes won't meet mine. His mouth is twisted into a rueful smile, an attempt to shelter a more vulnerable feeling, a soft underbelly he rarely shows.

"Do you know what he's referring to, Molly?" Evelyn asks.

I nod again, a wave of shame crashing over me. I force myself to speak: "I said something like *I wish I could escape and come over right now.*"

Stewart exhales again. "It was that word. *Escape.* It made me feel . . . I don't know . . ."

My voice falters, coming out as a whisper: "I didn't mean I wanted to escape from you. It's more like wanting to escape from my role. As a wife. As a mother."

"Well, it hurt," he says simply. "It hurt a lot."

I turn from Stewart to Evelyn and see the sympathy on her face. Sympathy for Stewart, I'm sure. Something about this feels unjust. Am I not allowed to desire an escape? A sudden blast of anger burns my shame to ash.

"I know it hurts. You've been escaping from us for years." I feel a storm brewing in my chest, and now my voice rumbles, an ominous thunder. "It's like you have some sort of allergy to domesticity. You've *never* wanted to be home. And *I* was the one—for years and years and years—who did all the bedtimes and school pickups, and the cooking and the cleaning and the laundry, and shuttling the kids to birthday parties and after-school activities and doctor's appointments. And *you* said you had to work. But now you seem to have time for other women, and one woman in particular. So yeah, maybe it's *my* turn for an escape."

The storm blows out as quickly as it blew in, leaving me shaking. I have an urge to apologize, to backpedal. But no. This is what I've worked on with Mitchell, right? Letting go of Straight-A Molly? Allowing myself to feel anger?

Evelyn lets silence envelop us for a few moments. Then she turns to Stewart. "Is there some truth to what Molly's saying?" I wait for his denial, but instead he nods. Evelyn continues: "Is there a reason you've avoided being at home?"

For a fleeting moment, I dismiss this line of inquiry as ridiculous. My rage is justified, ironclad in its resistance to cross-examination. For over a decade, I have been the self-sacrificing wife and mother. What could Stewart possibly say in his own defense? But then Stew leans back against the couch. I see the heaviness in his body, and I realize he has an answer. I hold my breath.

"I feel like I can never please you. For a long time now. Ever since Daniel was born. Everything I do is wrong."

The room seems to tip over and resettle upside down. I become aware of my folded arms, my pursed lips, the self-righteousness oozing out of my pores.

The rest of the session goes by in a haze. Evelyn questions Stewart about the weeks following Daniel's birth, when Stewart's father got sick with pneumonia and died within a matter of days. I listen as he untangles the threads of stressors during the months that followed. We had a new baby, and this was challenging enough. On top of it, Stewart was grieving, depressed. He guesses that I didn't have enough energy to take care of both Daniel's and his needs, so I dedicated myself to Daniel's. And he's right. I figured the best thing I could do for Stewart was to take on as much of the parenting load as I possibly could. And I did.

Evelyn's and Stewart's voices meld into a backdrop for new questions forming within me. At what point was Stewart ready—perhaps even *needing*—to come back into the fold of our newly formed family? When could I have relinquished some of my control, my notion of the "right" way to feed and diaper and bathe and soothe our baby son? When had my compassion for Stewart transformed into resentment, making him feel he wasn't doing enough, even as I insistently took over every domestic and parenting task?

"I know this is hard," says Evelyn, "but you two have done great work today. You've pushed through surface feelings to get at some old history. It's a lot to take in all at once, so let me see if I can summarize the big things I heard today."

I concentrate on looking at Evelyn, hoping she can throw us a lifeline.

"Molly, you're feeling stuck in the role of being a wife and mother and all that those roles entail. So being with Karl offers you a respite from that. And, Stewart, you've been feeling like you can't live up to Molly's standards for you. That you're constantly disappointing her. And maybe being with Kiwi is appealing to you because her standards are easier to meet. Because you don't have to do any of the difficult things with her—like raising children or building a life together."

I look at Stewart, and we nod at Evelyn in unison. It all sounds neat and tidy when she says it, but my head is aching, and Stewart looks like he's been hit by a truck.

"So now what do we do?" I ask.

"There are no magical answers," Evelyn says. "In some ways, open marriage is a joint adventure, something you're doing together. But at the same time, your outside relationships are individual explorations. And there are risks. You don't want to head off into the wilderness without knowing how to find your way home. You two need to figure out how to stay truly connected through all this. And that," she concludes, standing up to signal the end of our session, "is easier said than done."

I'm afraid to look at Stew as we walk out of the office, but I grab his hand and hold it as we ride down the elevator in silence, each absorbed in our own thoughts.

Evelyn is right. This is not just *our* journey as a couple—it is Stewart's, and it is mine. We can't possibly know where these paths will lead, or if they will even lead us back to each other. But I feel a larger force pulling me along.

No, I don't want to lose Stewart.

And I don't want to lose myself, either.

CHAPTER 12

ON SATURDAY, I'M ON my bed folding laundry again as I talk to my mom on the phone. I've noticed a new restlessness in my hands, a need to put them to constant use. Most of the time, there is plenty to keep them occupied: emails to type, dishes to wash, bills to sort. But when I'm waiting in line somewhere or walking down the street—particularly now that Nate no longer needs or wants to hold my hand—my thumb taps against the other digits in turn. Back and forth, like I'm trying to remove a sticky substance from my fingertips. It's a subconscious motion, one that abates only when I give my hands a clear task. Folding laundry has become my go-to activity for phone calls.

"Mom . . . ," I say, after our routine pleasantries have been exchanged. Since the session with Evelyn, I've been working on a question for my mother, a way to distill essential information from the confused muddle in my brain. "Can I ask you something? It's kind of a tough question, and I don't know if this is the right time."

"No time like the present!" says my mother, the Queen of Jolly Aphorisms.

"Did you ever really believe any of that stuff Mahikari taught about healing and divine light and everything?" I blurt, then try to soften the question: "I'm so relieved you're willing to take this Parkinson's drug—but there was a time when you wouldn't even let me take Sudafed."

She's quiet on the other end of the line. "I still feel awful about that."

"It's okay, Mom," I say, stifling any anger that threatens to surface. What would be the point? "I guess what I want to know is, did you join Mahikari because of Jim? Or did you want to join for yourself?"

"Oh my," my mother says, laughing nervously. "That *is* a tricky question."

"I'm just trying to understand. I mean, I remember you doing tai chi and stuff like that." I can picture my mother in the living room with her friend Ivy, wearing leotards and tights, moving like twin statues come to life, their arms cutting through the air so slowly it made me want to run out the door. "That was kinda normal, I guess—for the seventies. But what drew you to Mahikari?"

"Well," she says. "At that time of my life, I was searching. Seeking something larger than myself. And Jim was part of it, but certainly not all of it."

"How so?" I say, sitting up straighter. The same pair of jeans remains unfolded in my lap, and my fingers have resumed their compulsive thrumming.

"How do I explain it?" she asks herself. I wait until she continues: "Did I tell you that Dad and I used a code name for Jim? Before the two of them met each other, at least."

"What kind of code name?"

My mother giggles on the other end of the line, an echo of the laughter Jim used to summon from her depths.

"Jesus Christ."

"Seriously?" Now I'm laughing, too. "Why?"

"It started because he had the part of Jesus Christ in a play. But it was more than that. He was like a spiritual guide to me."

I take this in. "And Dad also called him that? I mean, he saw Jim as having that role in your life, too?"

"Oh, yes. Dad thought Jim was very important for me. Both sexually and spiritually," she adds.

I grimace at the idea of my father using the word *sexual* to describe my mother. A wave of sympathy for Daniel washes over me. No one ever wants to think of their parents that way. But I'm also fascinated. Does this mean my father felt true *compersion*? That he was happy for my mother to be on her own journey—one that involved sex as well as the spirit—apart from him?

"And then, of course, there was Buddha."

I'm snapped out of my thoughts. "Buddha?"

"Well, that was another code name, of course."

I think back to the conversation I had with my mother after everything ended with Matt: *Oh, sweetheart. There will be more.*

"And who was Buddha?" I ask.

She's quiet for a beat. "You really don't know?"

"AND WAS SHE RIGHT? Did you know who Buddha was?" Mitchell asks a few days later, after I catch him up. Now that Stew and I are seeing Evelyn, my sessions with Mitchell are only once a month. Mitchell has already slowed me down several times, assuring me we have plenty of time. I'm amazed when I glance at the clock and see that in fifteen minutes, I've told him the backstory on couples therapy, Karl, and my mother. I even remembered to share the compliment Daniel gave Stewart and me at our family's celebration of his fourteenth birthday: *You guys are the perfect balance of not boring but not crazy.*

"I didn't know right away," I say. "But I pushed my mom to tell me, and then it all made sense."

Buddha was a sensei of aikido—a martial art with deeper spiritual roots than either karate or judo—and on my mother's first visit with Jim to the Mahikari dojo, Buddha gave her his card, inviting her to come to his other dojo, for aikido. My mother went, donned a *gi,* and started as a white belt. Sometimes I went to the children's class, which mostly involved tumbling around on the floor. I'd met Buddha, but I barely remembered his real name.

"My mom told me Buddha had health problems—something with his kidneys. So Jim was the one who first told her about Mahikari, but Buddha actually *asked* her to become a member. He wanted her to be able to give him divine light or whatever. And on top of that"—I take a deep breath—"Buddha told her to stop seeing Jim. He was okay with my mother being married, but the idea of her having another lover made him too jealous. So she did what he wanted. She stopped seeing Jim—in a romantic way, at least."

"And what does that bring up for you?" Mitchell asks, reaching for his pad of paper. He must see an insight coming. I'm afraid of what it might be.

"Well, it makes me question if my mother ever did *anything* for herself," I say. "I mean, seeing other men was my father's idea. And then this whole spiritual quest of hers was driven by the men she was involved with. Even her names for them: Jesus Christ and Buddha. Like they're divine beings or something. Like the men have all the answers, and she's just following them. Like a disciple."

Mitchell nods encouragingly as he scribbles notes.

"So I'm wondering if that's the source of the 'repressed rage' she told me about." I pause. Mitchell stops writing and looks at me, waiting.

"It freaks me out a little. I thought her sexual freedom was the one release valve she had. But what if it was just, I don't know, an illusion of freedom?" My tears are rising again.

"And I'm guessing," says Mitchell, looking at the magical place on the ceiling that gives him all the answers, "that you're worried about the same thing? That open marriage is giving you an illusion of freedom, too?"

I nod, reaching for the tissues, my constant companion in therapy. "I mean, Karl asked me to stop seeing other men, too."

"Not exactly," says Mitchell. "I thought he said that your dating other people made him jealous, but did he really ask you to stop?"

"No," I say. "I guess he didn't. I think it was the right decision for me, too, but I'm having trouble trusting my instincts now. What if I'm just doing what Stewart and Karl *want* me to do?"

"That's a very important question to ask yourself."

I look at the ceiling now. Why can Mitchell find so many insights up there, but I never can? "And there's another thing. Martina wants to meet me. And I'm not sure how I feel about that. I guess it's no big deal. Plus, I know it will make Karl happy if we get along with each other."

"Okay," says Mitchell, returning to his pad of paper. "And what's on the other side of that answer? What does your gut say?"

"It makes me nervous. I feel like everything will be more complicated. We have a great system now. I go to their apartment while she's at her girlfriend's place, and there's no awkwardness around it."

Mitchell nods without looking up, continuing to write.

"But *The Ethical Slut* says it's a good idea to meet your partner's partners. That we're likely to imagine the worst, but it's usually fine. And I *am* kind of curious."

Mitchell smiles at me, remaining silent.

"So you're not going to weigh in on what I should do?" I ask.

"There's no right answer, Molly," he says. "Just pay attention to your own internal cues. And now, shall we set up our next appointment?"

THAT NIGHT, A HEAVY snowstorm descends on New York and interrupts my anxious musings about Karl, Martina, my mother,

Stewart, Kiwi. With school canceled for both kids and sidewalks to shovel, I'm adequately distracted.

In the afternoon, Nate begs me to take him sledding in Prospect Park. As we plod toward Seventh Avenue through the drifts, I feel my phone buzz in the pocket of my snow pants. Hoping it's a text from Karl, I rip off a glove and dig through my layers to check.

Hallo, Molly! Are you enjoying the snow? As usual, his German diction makes me smile.

Yes! I'm taking Nate to the sledding hill now! I reply, typing with one finger.

We're going sledding, too! Martina's friend has children and invited us! We'll meet you at the top of the hill!

So many exclamation points. So little time to process the words they punctuate. My mind goes as numb as my extremities, and I slow my pace.

"C'mon, Mom!" shouts Nate, urging me forward.

Within ten minutes, we reach the hill. At six foot three and 250 pounds, Karl will be hard to miss, but still, I survey the surroundings so as not to be caught off guard. Nate is too excited to notice my distraction and darts away to find his friends. I pull off my gloves to type another message to Karl—*We're here!*—and as I hit Send, I see him waving to me from across the snowy landscape. I guess that the shorter of the two women by his side is Martina. I wave weakly back.

As they approach, Martina's friend and her kids peel off. I take a few steps forward and stop. Can I hug Karl? Or should I hug Martina? Frozen with indecision, I keep my arms firmly at my sides, smiling and nodding idiotically at them both. Karl grabs me up in an embrace and kisses me on both cheeks in his European way. Martina looks at us with what I want to believe is a natural Resting Bitch Face, and I quickly go in to hug and double-kiss her, too, trying to make every interaction equitable. She receives me stiffly.

"Hi, Martina," I say, hoping the cold weather masks my flushed face and mild tremors. "It's great to finally meet you!"

Martina lets out a short laugh that sounds like a scoff. "You too. Karl talks about you a lot." She shoots him a sideways glance.

I try to will Karl to wipe the grin off his face, but he goes on beaming at us both. "This is so crazy! It is like seeing your teacher at the grocery market!" He laughs at his own joke.

From behind Karl, I spot Nate running toward me. He flings himself into the middle of our triangle and breaks the awkwardness. "Mom, can you watch me go down the hill?" he pants.

"Okay," I say, hiding my delight at this interruption. "But first say hello to my friends."

"Hi!" He waves noncommittally. "Let's go, Mom!"

Attaboy, I think as Nate leads me away. "Bye, Karl! Bye, Martina! It was so nice meeting you!"

"Likewise," she slurs.

"Good-bye!" shouts Karl, still beaming as if everything is not only okay but positively grand.

The next two hours are painful. I try to keep my focus on Nate and his *Watch me!* sledding tricks, but my attention keeps wandering back to Martina. She hates me. That much is obvious. Right now, she's probably telling Karl she wants him to break up with me. And then I'll be alone while Stewart gallivants around New Jersey with his new Kiwi girlfriend. I keep one nervous hand inside my pocket so as not to miss the all-important *bzzzzz,* signaling a text from Karl that will reveal my fate.

Finally, as Nate and I trudge back home in the dusk, it comes. *Martina is so mad at me,* I read. My breath catches in my throat.

And then: *It is because I didn't tell her how hot you are. She was unprepared.*

I look down at my snowsuit-clad body, complete with bib, which gives me a figure approximating the Michelin Man's. A scarf is wrapped around the bottom half of my face, as it has been the entire afternoon, and my hair is tucked up into a hat framed by an enormous hood. How can she think I'm hot? She couldn't even see me.

She wants the three of us to get together this week. Is that okay?

Sure, I write back quickly to avoid thinking about it. *That would be awesome.*

THE NEXT TIME I see Martina is thus planned as an outing for the three of us: a meetup at a bar for trivia night. Choosing an outfit for the evening throws me into a tailspin. Does Martina *want* me to be sexy? Or will that threaten her? I decide on a sweater dress that's cute but not too form-fitting and start my slow walk to the bar to meet them.

They're already inside when I get there. Martina stands up and, to my surprise, wraps me in a tight hug. She's wearing a long, slinky dress with horizontal stripes I could never get away with. On her, however, it looks stunning. She has large breasts and a small waist—and has clearly birthed zero children. Despite the cold weather, her curly hair is still wet from the shower.

"You smell good," I say without thinking. *Oh God,* I panic internally. *Now she'll think I'm some kind of hair-sniffing weirdo.*

But her face lights up at the compliment, and I feel a wave of understanding: *Feed Martina's ego, and all will be well.*

Martina slides into the booth next to Karl, and I take a seat across from them. When Karl reaches under the table and squeezes my knee, I bat his hand away, keeping my face neutral. Doesn't he understand what's at stake here?

"We need a team name," says Martina.

"How about the Polyamorists?" says Karl with a grin.

Martina waves her hand, dismissing the suggestion. "I was

thinking of Two Smart Women and Karl." She smirks at me, and I laugh uncomfortably. Karl has told me that Martina is very proud of her advanced degrees, and since Karl didn't go to college—he didn't even get his high school diploma, choosing to pursue photography instead—she likes to lord her intellect over him. But this doesn't feel like harmless teasing. There's something aggressive behind her words. Or maybe I'm just reading too much into it?

"I will go get us drinks," says Karl. "I think I know what *both* of you will like." He laughs in his lighthearted, goofy way, and I smile at Martina, trying to gauge her reaction to Karl's emphasis on the two of us as a unit. Her Resting Bitch Face returns. It's like I'm back in middle school and have landed a seat at the mean girls' table. I need to make myself small enough to avoid scrutiny.

"So Karl tells me you skipped a grade," she says. "Are you a genius or something?"

Oh shit, I think. *I really am back in middle school.*

"Definitely not!" I hope my expression conveys the absurdity of this idea.

"Karl seems to think you are," she says. Her eyes let me know she's far from convinced.

"That's just because he doesn't speak English," I say.

She bursts out laughing and puts her hand on my arm. "Haha! That's so true!" she snorts. I'm playing a game invented by twelve-year-old girls: making fun of others as a bonding rite.

Karl comes back with our drinks and smiles at the scene before him: his fiancée yukking it up with his girlfriend, everyone having a great time. Does he know that it's a façade? I follow Martina's lead, pretending to laugh along with her as she pokes fun at Karl—about his "poor" English, his weight, his lack of a steady paycheck. I feel vaguely troubled, but he doesn't seem to mind. Maybe this is simply Martina's way of dealing with her own insecurities? In any case, I'm grateful the focus isn't on me.

But when the trivia questions begin, I mistakenly step into the spotlight. I know more answers than Martina does. And once my competitive streak has been roused, it's hard to squelch.

What year did the United States boycott the Olympics?

"That was 1980!"

In Lewis Carroll's poem, what creatures do the walrus and carpenter eat?

"Oysters!"

Who was Mark McGwire's rival in the home run race of 1998?

"Sammy Sosa!"

It isn't until round three that I notice her irritation. I make excuses for what I know.

"Oh, I'm older than you, Martina," I say, trying flattery. "Were you even alive in 1980?

"I was an English teacher after all. I'd better know Lewis Carroll!

"My dad is a Cubs fan. I swear that's the only baseball question I could possibly answer."

She's also had four drinks to my two—and maybe a few more before I arrived. Her earlier demeanor—which I tried to believe was upbeat—has now turned decidedly sour. I start feigning ignorance at every question, and we leave before the final round.

The three of us stand outside for several awkward moments as I devise my exit strategy. I go to hug Martina good-bye first. Then, to my surprise, Karl leans in to hug Martina, too.

"I'm going to walk Molly home, okay?" he says lightly.

Oh shit.

"You don't have to do that," I sputter. "I can get home on my own."

"No, he'll walk you," says Martina with a tight smile. "That's clearly what he wants to do." She does an abrupt about-face and starts stumbling away in the other direction.

"She's upset, Karl," I shout-whisper. "I'm going to leave. You go home with her."

"No, please. Just wait here. She is fine. I promise. Let me only talk to her. I will be right back." And with a few lumbering steps he's caught up with Martina on the corner.

I busy myself with my phone and attempt to eavesdrop, but I can't trust the snatches of conversation that reach my ears. *You can go fuck her right now for all I care,* I hear or imagine I hear. Should I wait where Karl left me or turn and go? *This is how it will end,* I think. Martina will force him to break up with me, and I'll have to start dating all over again. I can't do it. I'll tell Stewart that I tried as hard as I could, but I just can't do open marriage anymore.

The next moment, Karl is striding toward me, smiling broadly.

"Everything is fine," he announces. "Let's go."

I give him a disbelieving look, but he takes my elbow and steers me forward. We walk the first block in silence, and then he speaks: "She really likes you. She is just angry at me. She gets like that when she drinks."

"But she's angry at you for walking me home! You should've left with her!" I protest.

"No, no, that's not it," he says, pushing his glasses up the bridge of his nose. "If I tell you, do you promise not to get upset?"

"Um, okay," I say, already breaking my promise.

"She is jealous. Not that I am with you, but that you are with me." I can feel his gaze, but I don't turn to meet it. "I think she might feel better if we could . . . you know . . . all sleep together. But only if you want to. No pressure."

My mind returns to our old apartment on the Upper West Side, the year before Stewart and I got married. After our second visit to Le Trapeze, I decided I was done with sex clubs. We pivoted instead to the idea of a good old-fashioned threesome. In college, and immediately after, I'd had a few crushes on female friends, though I was never sure if my attraction to women was truly sexual. But when Stewart told me that his ex-girlfriend Wild Wendy—the name differentiated her from Boring Wendy, whom he'd also dated—wanted to meet me, I started to wonder. I knew from Stew's stories that Wild Wendy preferred women to men. I also knew that she was outrageous enough to make Stewart uninterested in anything beyond sex. Maybe an FFM threesome would be a safe way to test the depths of my bisexuality.

"You're exactly her type," Stew told me as he fondled my breasts and fingered me in anticipation.

But the reality of our night with Wendy turned out to be different from my fantasies. I expected sex with a woman to be soft and gentle—that a woman's hands on my body would know exactly what to do, that it would feel almost like masturbation. But it never occurred to me that a woman's touch would be a turn*off.* Yet that's the way I felt. Her lips were too yielding. Her hands were too small. I licked her breasts, and by the force of some complex that was not covered in Psych 101, they tasted like *milk* to me. I didn't mind looking at Wendy's naked body for its aesthetic value, but I had no interest in caressing it. Instead, the two of us took turns sucking Stewart's cock until he came. Afterward, Wild Wendy lay in our double bed with us—talking incessantly about the latest job she'd been fired from—until I yawned dramatically and suggested Stewart hail her a cab.

Maybe a threesome with Karl and Martina will be different, I wonder.

"Let me think about it," I tell him.

"That's all I want you to do," he says with a grin.

THAT WEEKEND, I DRIVE to a teachers' conference at the Marriott Boston in Quincy. The miles fly by. On long drives by myself,

I usually stop frequently to avoid falling asleep at the wheel. But now my mind feels hyperalert, a beehive of activity. My thoughts will not, cannot stray from Karl—and, of course, Martina. I again feel her eyes looking me up and down when I arrived at the bar. I remember her inscrutable, tight smile when Karl announced his intention to walk me home. And then I imagine myself telling Karl that I don't think a threesome is a good idea, that I'm afraid things will get too complicated, too messy. I see his round, boyish face clouded in disappointment at my refusal. Next, I imagine saying yes, and his face lighting up at the idea of the three of us in bed together. Despite my reservations, my body tingles as I consider the thrill of giving this to him. *I just might enjoy myself, too,* I think. *Wasn't Martina's own girlfriend "straight" before they started dating? Maybe Martina has a magic touch.* Round and round my thoughts go, swirling themselves into a rolling boil.

The Marriott Boston is a horrible misnomer, as Quincy is nowhere near Boston, and alone in my remote hotel room, I find no respite from my anxiety. I text Karl to see if he can talk and get what feels like a dismissive response: *Sorry. I'm with Martina. Can't text now.* I know Stewart is on a date with Kiwi. Prior to our last session with Evelyn, we agreed to "give each other space" while out with other people. This was an idea I fully sanctioned, as it allowed me to turn off my ringer whenever I was with Karl. But now I think of Evelyn's warning: "Make sure you know how to find your way home." I don't think I can make it through the evening without Stew. And so I text him, trying to infuse my desperation with a bit of humor: *I'm fantasizing about checking myself into the nearest psych ward. Can I call you please?*

My phone rings almost immediately. "What's up, baby?" he asks.

Hearing the concern in his voice sends me into convulsions of sobs.

"Take it easy, honey," he says gently. "Tell me what's going on."

"I'm so sorry I'm bothering you while you're on a date," I wail.

"It's okay, really. Kiwi totally gets it. She just stepped out so you and I can talk privately."

Stepped out, I think. Of their hotel room, of course. But then the jealousy that this image evokes transforms itself into gratitude: *Kiwi gets it. Thank God he's dating someone who's open, too.*

"I feel like I'm losing my mind," I say. "I don't know why it's such a big deal to me, but I don't know what to do!"

"About what?" says Stew.

"About what?!" I shriek. "The threesome! I told you yesterday—Martina wants to have a threesome, and I don't know if it's a good idea."

"Right," says Stew. I suspect he's suppressing laughter. "You realize this isn't a life-or-death decision, right? Do it if you want to, but it sounds to me like you don't. And I don't think I have to remind you: the night we spent with Wendy was awesome for me, but you weren't that into it."

"I know, I know," I say. "Mitchell says I need to pay attention to my gut. But my gut is so confused. I hate not knowing what to do!"

"Okay, my Indecisive One," he says, "let's start with some deep breaths." Stew breathes with me for a while and I start to feel better. "Remind me not to vote for you if you ever run for president, okay?"

I laugh. "Okay. I should let you go." I've almost forgotten that he's on a date. That he's not fully mine tonight.

As if he's read my mind, Stew says, "Tell you what. I want you to find something really stupid to watch on TV. The dumber the better. And I'm going to call you back in fifteen minutes to check on you. Okay?"

"You don't have to do that," I say unconvincingly.

"I know I don't have to. I want to. You're my wife. I love you.

And I don't want to have to drive to Boston to pick you up from the asylum tomorrow."

I laugh again. "And Kiwi won't mind?"

"She won't mind. She wants you to feel better, too."

"Okay, thanks," I say.

"Fifteen minutes," Stew repeats. "And you'd better be watching something idiotic."

"Got it."

I put down my phone and pick up the remote. Fifteen minutes later, I'm watching *Press Your Luck* on the Game Show Network when Stew calls again.

"All good?"

"All good," I say, turning up the volume so he can hear the contestants shout, "No Whammies!"

"Perfect," he says. "I love you, baby. I'll keep my ringer on in case you need to talk again."

"Thanks, Stewbie. I love you, too."

I fall asleep with the TV on and my phone in my hand.

THE NEXT DAY, AFTER fulfilling the bare minimum of my conference obligations, I drive home. Without any place to direct it, my suppressed anxiety starts to crystallize into an action plan that is almost manic in nature.

I know what I have to do. Karl and Martina and I will have a threesome. But only once. That evening, I tell Stew my plan, running the words together and barely stopping to breathe.

"I'm going to go over there, but just for a couple of hours. No, an hour and a half. And afterward, you need to meet me for a drink at the Dram Shop or someplace close by so I can process it. And that will give me an excuse to leave at a certain time. Okay? Can you do that for me? I'm going to text him now."

Stew looks at me, choosing his words with care, trying to slow down this runaway train disguised as his wife. "Are you *sure* you want to do this? I thought you weren't into women."

"I have to," I tell him. "Otherwise I'm going to keep obsessing about what will happen!" My logic is tenuous, but I need to believe it's rock-solid. I look at Stewart, willing him to back me up. He opens his mouth to speak but lets out a sigh instead.

"Do what you want, I guess," he says, throwing up his arms.

This is not the endorsement I crave.

THE PLANNING PROCESS FOR my ménage à trois is about as sexy as organizing a school fundraiser. First, to create adequate distance between my sexy self and my "mom" self, I arrange sleepovers for both Daniel and Nate—which means I'll need to reciprocate by hosting two of their friends the following weekend. Second, I choose what I'll wear. But instead of being decadent and fun, this feels like an impossible riddle. How do I dress up for Martina but not outshine her? In addition to an outfit, I have to pick out a bra and panties, pluck the errant hairs around my nipples without causing unsightly bumps, groom my bush. The tasks seem endless.

As I get ready to leave, I interrogate Stewart about my appearance.

"What do you think?" I ask him. "Or, more importantly, what do you think *she'll* think?"

"You look great, baby," he says. His eyes convey the same doubt that's been there since I first mentioned this whole idea. But he's trying a slightly different angle now. "The main thing is, you need to relax. I mean, I'm just spitballing here, but maybe you could try to *enjoy* yourself? 'Cause if you can't do that, I really don't understand the point."

He's right, of course. But I've already come this far. I'm at the edge of the Rubicon. Instead of admitting the truth—that I don't want to have a threesome with Karl and Martina, that I'm only doing this because it feels like a requirement for dating Karl at all—I put on the sunniest smile I can muster and tell Stew the same lie I'm telling myself: "All right, I'll enjoy myself! And I'll meet you at the Dram Shop at nine o'clock. Maybe get there a little early just in case?"

"I'll be there," he says in a resigned tone. He opens his arms for a hug. "I'll be there for whatever you need." I can't let myself relax enough to sink into him, but I inhale deeply, trying to gather in his essence as fortification.

I resist the urge to text Karl on my walk to his apartment. *No, their apartment,* I correct myself. My chance for one-on-one communication has passed, and the last thing I want is for Karl to share my doubts and insecurities with Martina. I've picked up two bottles of Oyster Bay sauvignon blanc—Martina's favorite, according to Karl. I hope that downing a glass will cure the paralysis of nerves that has locked me inside myself like a suit of armor.

But then as I ring the doorbell and see Karl at the end of the hall, walking toward me with a grin on his face, something shifts. My body is still made of iron, but I'm surprised by how fluidly it moves. And then I realize: this body is not me. I control it, but the true me is safely tucked away inside. There is nothing to fear.

"Hi there," I watch myself say to Karl. "I brought some wine."

I hand him the bag and walk past him, entering the apartment first. I smell the candles, hear the music. These sensory cues are reminders of the other me, the me who so enjoys coming to Karl's apartment, revels in letting down my defenses and allowing him to take care of me. But tonight, I'm someone else.

Martina is sitting on the couch, flipping idly through one of Karl's photography books. She smiles at me with one side of her mouth. I sit next to her—close—and hug her tightly. She isn't wearing a bra, and I feel her breasts against mine through her sweater. I note this sensation without assigning it meaning. It is neither good nor bad. Martina has breasts. My body also has breasts.

"I love your sweater," I hear myself say, as I keep my hand on her back, stroking the material. "It's so soft."

"Thanks," she says. She looks at me quizzically, surprised by my forwardness. I pull my hand back and remember, as if they are director's notes from a previous rehearsal—*Let Martina be in charge. She wants you to succumb to her. Don't overdo it.* Every move I make feels easier when I view it not with my eyes, but through the wide-angle lens hovering above this scene.

Karl comes in holding two glasses of wine. He hands one to me and takes a sip from the other before handing it to Martina. *See what Karl did there?* says my Inner Director. *That was a subtle cue that they are the primary couple, and you are the visitor. Follow their lead.*

I wait, sipping my wine and shaping my face into an expression of eager willingness. Karl is to my left on the couch, Martina to my right. They exchange a glance, and then Karl asks, as he did the first time we slept together, with just the slightest shift of pronoun, "May we undress you?"

I nod. Karl takes my glass from me, then moves my hair to the side to unzip my dress. Martina looks at me, smiling, and as Karl unclasps my bra, she pulls her sweater off and I see the perfection of her breasts up close. Inside my lockbox body, I regard the difference between her breasts and mine with a clinician's detachment. I have nursed two children; she has not. But even before I gave birth, my right side was a cup size bigger than my left, and my breasts have always stubbornly refused to meet each other halfway. For me, cleavage is an effect to be achieved with uncomfortable bras rather than a natural state. Martina, meanwhile, displays symmetrical scoops of peach ice cream, dotted with two semi-ripe cherries.

Seeing her breasts makes the hidden me squirm self-consciously, but only for a moment. Karl leans against one arm of the couch as Martina faces me from the other end. He is massaging my lopsided breasts with his large hands, and I relax back into my role. Martina leans in from stage right to kiss me, and I'm relieved to discover that she does not taste like milk. To confirm, I lower my head and taste each peach sundae in turn. She doesn't taste like anything at all, I note. My action sequence has the desired effect, and she begins to moan.

"Shall we go to bed?" asks Karl. I nod again, afraid to break the spell of our stage chemistry with spontaneous dialogue.

I stand up and wait as Karl removes my tights and panties, then takes off his own pants and shirt. Martina kisses me again, pushing her entire body against mine, and leads me by the hand to the bedroom. I note the clock on the kitchen wall. I need to be at the Dram Shop in fifty-seven minutes.

In their room, I put my hands and mouth on Martina in places I am expected to put them, and I let her do the same to me. Karl takes on a supporting role, touching me more than he touches Martina, which I hope is in the approved script. With her small hands, I let Martina bring me to orgasm—not entirely a performance, except for the volume of my screams—and I watch as she locks eyes with Karl and plunges her fingers into his mouth, letting him taste me. This feels like a cue, and I sit up, hoping I look sufficiently disheveled.

"Oh my God," I say. "That was amazing, Martina." I kiss her on the mouth, lingering for effect, and then I deliver my lines: "Stewart is expecting me soon. I promised him I wouldn't stay out late so he doesn't get too jealous."

I stretch dramatically and gather up my clothing from the living room. I go to the bathroom to pee and stay there to get dressed. I don't want to be pulled back into this scene.

Once I'm safely clothed, I wave coquettishly from the doorway as they lie naked on the bed. "Good-bye, you two." I don't register their response. I am out the door, on my way to Stewart. As I walk, I'm aware that my body is still not quite mine. But it's over.

Stewart is sitting at the bar at the Dram Shop, a glass of pinot noir reserving my place next to him.

"So how was it?" he asks as I take off my coat and perch on the stool. He already knows how it was, of course. He knew how it would go before it even happened.

"It was fun!" I chirp, fooling neither of us.

Stew puts his hand on the back of my neck and massages it gently. I feel his touch and breathe, starting to return to myself. I'm so glad my husband knows where I hide the key to the lockbox.

THE NEXT DAY, I receive a series of texts from Karl:

Martina and I had such a good time spoiling you last night.

It was so hot to see you two together.

Martina says I am not to change the sheets.

I feel a deep-seated uneasiness and respond with guarded enthusiasm: *I'm glad. . . . Me too. . . . Mmm . . .* The threesome has been checked off the to-do list, right? I've done what Martina asked for. My obligation is fulfilled.

That night, after washing the dishes and wrangling Nate to bed, I settle in to catch up on a few episodes of *Girls,* my mind finding rest in the gritty Greenpoint landscape. When my phone buzzes, I pick it up to see a text from a number I don't recognize.

Hi there. I stare at the three dots. *Karl just fucked me so well, but all I could think about was you.*

Panic and dread rise up in me, vying for the constricted space in my chest. I pause the TV. What should I say? I have to cut her off somehow, but carefully.

Oh hi, Martina, I write. *I've been thinking a lot about last night, too. Thanks so much for inviting me. Sleep well!* I add a couple of winky-face emojis for good measure and hit Send.

After turning off the TV, I lie awake for a long time.

The next morning, I wait until I'm sure Karl is at work and then I call, my hands shaking.

"Why did you give Martina my number?" I say in response to his "Hallo!"

"She asked me for it," he answers matter-of-factly, confused by the question.

CHAPTER 13

IN THE FOLLOWING WEEKS, I obsess over the drama of Karl and Martina as if it is the only story line in my life. In fact, that's what it has become. I see Martina only one more time. I stop by a gathering with their neighbors, just long enough to deliver another flirty performance and pretend to receive a call from Nate, ushering me home. But even Martina's absence is a presence. In every text exchange and every date with Karl—or even when I'm alone or with Stewart and the kids—she is always on my mind.

I know I'm slipping into dangerous territory when I cancel an appointment with Mitchell, then one with Evelyn. Only Stewart is privy to how lost I am inside this soap opera of my own making, how helpless I am to find a way out of it.

One morning, I give him the latest updates.

"So according to Karl, she understands that he and I need to have our own dates, but she wants to *watch* us have sex sometimes. I'm not comfortable with that being the new normal, though. So I suggested that if I *want* her to come in, we'll leave the bedroom door open, but otherwise, we'll leave it closed. And she freaked out! She told him she's never felt so disrespected in her life! Karl says not to worry about it, but I have no idea how to placate her. It feels impossible."

Stewart interrupts my monologue with an audible exhalation. "I'm going out with Kiwi tonight, okay?"

I pause. His flat statement hits me like a fall onto pavement. Shock protects me from hurt, at least for a few moments. "I thought you and I were hanging out tonight."

"Molly, I need a break." He turns away from me. "If I have to hear one more word about K-Mart, I'm going to lose my shit."

"Oh," I say.

He's right. Our time together has been poisoned, and any promise not to talk about Karl and Martina would be empty. I might as well swallow a bottle of ipecac and promise not to vomit.

But the hurt of Stewart needing a respite from me is only a small part of the pain that eats me from the inside out. I think I may have fallen in love with someone. And now I'm going to lose him.

"IS KARL BACK ON OkCupid?" Stewart asks a few nights later, in bed. I've been careful not to mention Karl and Martina, and I'm grateful that Stew is finally broaching the topic.

"No," I say. "Remember? He closed his account right after we started dating."

"Well, you might want to ask him again. He just 'liked' Kiwi."

"What?" I say, confusion morphing into panic. "How do you know?"

"She sent me a screenshot. Look."

Stewart hands me his phone, and there is Karl's face, filling the app's blue frame. As I stare, my brain attempts to make sense of what I'm seeing. Karl has lied to me. He's already looking for his next girlfriend to replace me. And Kiwi is the one who attracted his attention. She's going to take both my husband and my boyfriend and there is nothing I can do. I have let all of this happen, and now I'm powerless to stop it. The soft surface of the bed is too yielding, too accommodating to the brokenness inside me, and I roll off the edge and lie on the hard wooden floor. The crying begins as a low moan, but soon I'm wailing so violently I can barely speak.

"Why are you telling me this?" I ask Stew through my sobs. It's the only question I don't already know the answer to.

Stewart is still on the bed, and he peers down at me on the floor, unsure of how to deal with the wild animal before him. A wild, wounded animal is exactly what I feel myself to be—something unwieldy but vulnerable. Perhaps a baby hippo, huddled on the floor by the bed.

"Because I don't want you to get hurt," he says. "I'm trying to protect you. And Kiwi isn't going out with him or anything. She just thought you should know he's lying to you."

"If you want to protect me," I scream, "don't keep making me do this! Stop dating Kiwi and whoever else and just be with me. Don't you understand? I can't do this anymore!"

He reaches for me, but I won't let him touch me. I hold my hands over my ears like a child locked in a tantrum. I won't let him speak to me or comfort me, and I stay balled up on the floor in a rigid knot of pain. I wait until I hear Stew snoring before I crawl into bed, spent, still careful not to let his body touch mine.

THE NEXT MORNING, I awaken to an empty bedroom. Stewart has left for work early—to avoid me, I assume. This should sting, but my whole body is already a tender bruise. I sit holding my phone for several minutes. I need to confront Karl, but I don't trust myself to speak. I send a text instead. Rather than asking questions, I make declarative statements.

You reactivated your OKC profile. You "liked" Stewart's girlfriend.

The time that passes before his reply feels longer than the few minutes shown on my bedside clock. I jump when the phone vibrates and hold it to my chest before reading.

Martina must have done that. You know she likes straight women, so I let her go into the account as me.

I am not sure what to do with this information. The unapologetic mix of honesty and dishonesty. And what it means for me.

They are looking for new prey.

I'M ON AUTOPILOT, KEEPING my head down and dodging pedestrians as I walk the long avenues between Herald Square and Mitchell's office. My head pounds, but pain emanates from a place beyond the neurons in my skull. The pain is everywhere. Everything.

I've asked Mitchell for a double session and have written down an outline of events since my last appointment. I read them aloud from the Notes section of my phone, my voice cracking and tears leaking into a clutched tissue. When I'm done, I reach for the extra-large Dunkin' Donuts iced coffee I've brought and grip my forehead with the other hand, digging my thumb and ring finger into the temples.

"I see you have a migraine today."

"I've forgotten how it feels to *not* have a migraine."

Mitchell tents his fingers and looks at the ceiling. "The insidious thing about a migraine is how all-consuming it is. In fact, that may be a chief function of migraines. Or ulcers, backaches. Any debility associated with stress. In a way, the physical pain protects you from fully experiencing emotional pain."

"But I *am* feeling emotional pain," I say, starting to cry again to prove my point.

"Yes, I know," he says gently. "But you're attributing this pain to Karl, to Martina, to Stewart. I think the real source of your pain is much deeper."

"What do you mean?"

"Let's talk about Straight-A Molly. You said that during your threesome with Karl and Martina, you felt like your true self was hidden. Like you were performing a role. Do you think perhaps Straight-A Molly showed up that night?"

My lips go slack around the giant pink straw in my mouth. *Oh my God. He's right.* I nod.

He flips through his notebook and puts his finger on a page. "Ah, here's the list of Freedoms you made. September twenty-first, 2014. When we were 'Reassigning Straight-A Molly.' Remember?"

I nod. Even this small motion of my head makes me wince. *That was over a year and a half ago,* I think. *And I'm stuck in exactly the same place.*

"I think the most important one to recall right now is this: 'Freedom from pleasing others.' Do you agree?"

I stare dumbly at my Dunkin' Donuts cup. Clearly, it's my turn to make sense of all this. But I have no answers—just a single question.

"Why do I keep doing this?" I say, my voice emerging louder than intended. "Why can't I stop this stupid pleasing-everyone bullshit? I'm so FUCKING SICK OF MYSELF!" I'm screaming now, screaming from a place of anguish I cannot locate.

Mitchell sits across from me—still, gentle, waiting. I blow my nose and wait, too, wait for my muddled brain to produce a thought. And then a memory starts to emerge. I squeeze my eyes shut to let it form itself into words.

"What's coming up for you right now?" Mitchell asks me.

"I'm thinking of something my mom said when I first started dating Stewart."

"Yes?"

"She asked me, 'How do you feel about yourself when you're with him?' It was like a litmus test or something."

"And what was your answer?"

"I told her Stewart made me feel better about myself than anyone I'd ever known. I mean, William made me feel like shit. And Stew made me realize how love is *supposed* to feel. But . . ." My voice catches in my throat, strangled by the new round of sobs threatening to erupt.

"But what?"

I breathe. I need to get this out. "But the truth is, I've never felt good about myself," I say, "no matter who I'm with. The truth is I feel like shit about myself all the time." My tears are pouring out of me now, liquid pain. I've emptied the box of tissues on the side table, and Mitchell reaches for a second box from his desk and hands it to me.

"Molly, you're doing some wonderful work today," he says, with such enthusiasm that I laugh out loud.

"Yeah, I guess a two-tissue-box day earns a gold star, huh?"

"Not that I'm giving you an A," he says, smiling. "But you've reminded me of something else we talked about in a previous session. I think you've discovered the cause of the hole in your bucket."

I stop my sniveling and think about it. Yes, the hole in my bucket. The place where all my self-worth leaks away.

"What I'm hearing from you right now," he continues, "is that throughout your life, you've been looking outside of yourself—to your parents, to your kids, to Stewart, to Karl—for the validation and love you crave. But, Molly, you can't *receive* anyone else's love until you love yourself."

I sit up straighter, the pain in my head starting to diminish. I feel the truth in his words.

"Nobody else—not your mother, not your children, not your husband, not your lovers—will ever be able to fix this. Only *you* have the power to repair this hole."

As I leave Mitchell's office, I feel a new clarity in my vision. The migraine is gone, yes, but it's more, too. I need to take another break from dating. I need to date *myself.*

Without giving details, I text Stewart to tell him how much better I feel.

Yay! he writes. *Thank God for Mitchell!*

Then I text Karl. *Hi there. Can you and I make some time to talk?*

He doesn't write back.

I AM GHOSTED.

It's a term I didn't know before I entered the online dating world, but it's an apt description of what happens next. Karl evaporates into thin air—not responding to my texts or emails or phone calls—and I am left grieving as if he is dead. But I know he's alive.

In May, I see pictures on Facebook of Martina and Karl's wedding in Germany. Martina wears a wreath of flowers on her head and a lacy white dress. Karl stands next to her, his arm wrapped tightly around her waist, a goofy smile lighting up his face. Looking at the two of them together, I feel sure I spent more time thinking about Karl than he spent thinking about me. I was merely a pawn. Martina liked straight women. Karl's job was to bring them home to her. It was possible that Karl developed feelings for me, feelings he didn't expect, and because of that, Martina demanded a breakup. But if that's true, why would he refuse even one last text or email, a good-bye at the very least, something to let me feel less horribly used?

Maybe it's karma, I think. Matt was a prop in my marriage, and I was a prop in Karl's.

———

DURING THIS TIME, I feel like a hermit crab who has outgrown its shell. I'm running across the beach, naked and vulnerable, looking for refuge. I decide to reach out to Jessie. Our kids go to different schools and have grown apart, but this means the friendship has become entirely our own. We sit at her kitchen table, two mugs of coffee and a box of Kleenex between us. I catch her up on the saga of K-Mart—the shorthand makes her laugh—and thank her for giving me Mitchell's number all those years ago.

"I'm sorry I've been so out of touch," I say between eye dabs and nose blows. "I think I was avoiding you because I was afraid of what you'd say. And I knew you'd be right."

She laughs. "And what would I have been right about, exactly?"

"I don't know," I say. "Maybe that I was worrying too much about everyone else's needs and not paying enough attention to my own."

Jessie nods. She's going through a transition, too, having recently given up drinking. "What you're saying reminds me of something I heard at an AA meeting. It's the idea of being 'right-sized.' And I'm still trying to figure it out." She pauses and takes a sip of coffee.

"Can you give me an example?" I ask. I've missed these talks with Jessie. How we alternate between laughter and the deep questions of our inner lives.

"Well, like alcohol for me. Alcohol became too big a part of my life. I couldn't get through a day without it, so I'd spend way too much time thinking about when I would be able to drink. And then I'd drink too much, and the next morning would be shot because I felt terrible. I just couldn't manage to keep it right-sized—drinking always seemed to take over. So I decided I had to quit. I'm wondering if there's some wisdom there for you, too. Like, when Stewart got so upset because you couldn't stop talking about Karl and Martina. Or when you felt like you were losing your mind because you were obsessing over how to handle the whole situation."

I stop and think while we both sip our coffee. "Yeah," I say. "It totally fits. That relationship was definitely *not* right-sized."

"But that doesn't necessarily mean you should close your marriage," she says, surprising me. "God knows I wish I could drink moderately and not have to give it up. Maybe it's more something to ask yourself. Do you think you can make open marriage a 'right-sized' part of your life?"

It's a great question.

ONE EVENING, I'M HELPING Nate with a huge math packet he's supposed to complete by the last day of school. It's a scenario that regularly ends in tears—for both of us. I go up to my bedroom while Nate takes a break from the offending equations, and I unload my frustration on a pillow, pummeling it until I exhaust myself. Afterward, the migraine creeping around the edges of my awareness dissipates. I sit at my computer later that night, google *NYC women's boxing,* and find a women-only boxing class.

I sign up for the foundations clinic over the next four Saturdays. The first week, there are five of us, and by the last week, only one other woman and I show up. I have yet to land a single punch, but I've jumped rope, worked on my shuffle, and done hundreds of burpees. I'm excited to join the "real" class when the next session starts.

I've also fallen into a pleasant routine as I take the subway to and from the boxing gym. I keep several volumes of my mother's favorite magazine in my boxing bag—she gifted me a subscription last Christmas. It arrives monthly, filled with personal essays, poetry, and beautiful photographs. On the back of the June issue, I see info for a weekend writing retreat in North Carolina.

"Do you want to go?" I ask my mother over the phone. There's a pause on the other end.

"Really? How?"

"Dad could take you to the airport, and I'll meet you when your plane lands in Charlotte. We'll rent a car and a wheelchair for you, and we'll get a double room so I can help you get to the bathroom and stuff."

I can hear the tears in her voice. "Molly, I can't think of anything more wonderful."

In the week preceding the trip, we choose our sessions from the catalog of offerings. We agree to attend all the same workshops so she'll have me on hand. While she wants to work on her poetry, I plan to bring my guitar and do some songwriting. I'm looking forward to the trip, but Mitchell has warned me to watch out for Straight-A Molly.

"She will say yes to anything," he reminds me. "But True Molly is likely to feel resentful."

Sure enough, by the end of the first night—after collecting my mother from the airport, driving one hundred miles on foggy mountain roads, and maneuvering through a family-style dinner and the opening get-to-know-you session—I have a raging migraine. As I help my mom take off her compression socks and arrange her medication on the bedside table, I keep a smile on my face. I'm afraid to take Tylenol PM. I have to be able to hear her call if she needs me during the night.

I lie in bed, grimacing, the stiff pillow like a rock grinding against my skull. My mother is having such a wonderful time. I don't want to ruin it by letting her know how much pain I'm in. But through the throbbing, a memory surfaces, the words she said to me when I was ten years old and asked me to join Mahikari: *You would make me the happiest mother in the world.*

Have I ever stopped feeling the pressure to make her—or later

Stewart, my children, Karl—happy? To dutifully meet everyone's needs but my own?

How do I even figure out what my own needs are? my migraine asks me.

Spending the night with my mother is like having a newborn. She wakes me up only once, around one a.m., for help getting to the bathroom, but I remain on high alert, just as I used to wait for Daniel's or Nate's cries. I drift back to sleep as the first light of dawn appears through the flimsy curtains, and the next thing I know, I'm jarred awake by my mom's portable alarm clock. Six a.m.

She needs a full two hours to get ready for the day. The first step is taking her medication. After eight hours without it, her body is as limp as a puppet. It takes nearly thirty minutes for the pills to kick in, and then—with my help—she can make her way to the bathroom. But in the interim, none of her muscles do her bidding, including the ones that hold back urine.

"I'm so sorry you have to deal with this mess," she says, glancing down at her wet nightgown.

"It's okay, Mom," I say. "It's no big deal." And, in truth, it isn't. She wears an overnight Depend and sleeps on a disposable pad. All I have to do is throw these things in the garbage and put her nightgown in a plastic bag. But I see the embarrassment on her face and feel my own shame for forgetting to brighten my expression. Despite the pain radiating from my temples and the dull nausea that comes with it, I force a smile.

"Let's get you into a hot shower," I say with false cheer.

It turns out that two hours isn't enough. The dining hall is on the other side of the retreat center, and I push my mother across a pathway of resistant gravel, making it to breakfast half an hour late. Her anxiety is now triggered. She needs food with her second round of pills, and the first session is set to begin at nine.

"Don't worry, Mom," I say. "I'll settle you at a table and then I'll bring you something. How about oatmeal?"

"Thank you, sweetie," she says, glancing around nervously at the tables of chattering retreat-goers. I see the fear of small talk on her face.

I spot a half-filled table and approach with my sunniest face and a voice to match. "Good morning! I'm Molly, and this is my mother, Mary. May we join you?"

"Oh yes!" exclaims a plump woman with a long gray braid. As I park the wheelchair at the table, she reaches for my mother's hand. "Hello, Mary! We noticed you and Molly at the orientation last night. It's so lovely to watch the two of you together. Aren't you lucky to have a daughter like that by your side?"

My mother nods. "I couldn't do it without her!"

By the time I've served my mother and helped organize her pills, I've given up on a real breakfast for myself. I slip a banana into my bag and fill my travel mug with coffee. We're late to the first session, and then we miss the writing prompt because my mother has to pee again.

"I shouldn't have had that coffee," she whispers to me, shame-faced again.

The closest bathroom involves climbing three steps, so we wander the grounds, trying to find a restroom that's accessible by ramp, and end up back at the dining hall. It's a tight squeeze for two people and a wheelchair, so while my mother is on the toilet, I sit in her chair.

"Oh, Molly," my mom says, shaking her head sorrowfully. "You're missing everything because of me."

"It's okay, Mom," I say for maybe the tenth time that day. "You're the reason I'm here. I'm not missing anything." As the words leave my mouth, a pain stabs my brain. I can't help but wince.

"Oh, dear. Are you having a migraine?" she asks.

"Yes," I admit. "But don't worry about it. It'll pass."

We sit in silence for a moment. This is not unusual when my mother is on the toilet, and I assume she's concentrating on trying to "go."

"Have you heard of the oxygen mask theory?" she asks me.

I have. It's based on the instructions you get on a plane. When the cabin pressure falls, you're supposed to put on your own mask before helping others. I first learned this as a parenting concept at a Mommy & Me Yoga class I took when Daniel was nine months old. I understood the analogy in theory—that self-care is part of caring for others—but I never managed to practice much yoga while trying to breastfeed or chase a crawling baby.

"Yes," I say. "I'm not sure it's a very realistic idea."

"I've always struggled with it, too," says my mother with a sigh. "But I wonder if it's the root cause of your migraines. You're here trying to take care of me, and you can't get enough air for yourself."

I stare at her, astonished. "That's exactly what I figured out in therapy."

"Oh, that's so good!" my mother exclaims. She seems genuinely excited. "Your therapist must be wonderful."

"But it's not just about taking care of you," I say. "It's about everything I do." My voice drops off, and before I can stop myself, my eyes fill with tears.

"Oh, sweetie," my mother says. She reaches for the toilet paper, tears off a wad, and hands it to me. In the time it takes her to do this, I could have gotten six tissues for myself, but I let her complete the gesture. I let her take care of me in this small way.

"I honestly don't mind helping you on this trip, though," I say, guilt churning inside me as I snuffle and blow my nose. It would be more honest to say that I *wished* I didn't mind.

"Well, unfortunately, I don't see a way around it at this point," she says, looking down at herself, still sitting on the toilet with her pants around her ankles. She starts to giggle.

"You mean I shouldn't steal your wheelchair and leave you here?" I ask, chuckling along with her now.

"I suppose someone would find me," she says, laughing harder. "Eventually!"

We are both gasping for air as the sound of our hilarity fills the tiny bathroom. My mother clutches her chest, and I can see her, young and beautiful, holding the rotary phone as Jim sends her into similar spasms.

It takes several attempts, but once we catch our breath, my mother grabs my hand.

"I think there is no lovelier feeling than laughter through tears," she says. I squeeze her hand and nod my agreement.

We decide not to bother rushing back to the first session—especially once I realize I've forgotten my guitar.

"Let's go get it," says my mom. "The next workshop sounds perfect for songwriting." I'm excited about it, too. It's titled The Music of Writing, and the instructor who's leading it stood out among last night's introductions.

We leave the dining hall once again, and I push my mother through the insidious gravel in the direction of our room. I've broken into a sweat, wondering if all-terrain wheelchairs exist, when I hear a whirring sound behind me. I turn around and see a golf cart coming toward us along the path.

"Good morning, ladies!" It's the guy in charge of daily operations at the retreat center. He gave a short orientation at our opening meeting, telling us everything from the history of the land to the location of the recycling bins. He's a man of indeterminate age. His glasses and slender build give him the air of a professor—in sharp contrast to his work boots and rough hands. "Can I offer you a lift? Where are you headed?"

"Oh, that's really nice of you," I say. "But we're okay. I just forgot something in our room."

"Do you need to go to the room too, Mary? I'd be happy to put your chair in the back of this contraption and take you directly to your next session."

My mother's eyes widen in surprise. "How do you know my name?" she asks. "I'm embarrassed to say I can't remember yours."

"I never forget a pretty lady," he says. "I'm Chris. And don't be embarrassed. There were a lot of people who introduced themselves last night."

"Well," says my mother, straightening up, "I certainly won't forget you twice. And I would be delighted to have such a handsome escort!"

I watch this exchange in dumb horror. My mother is *flirting!*

"Well then, let's be on our way!" He offers his hand and helps my mom to the passenger side. She continues to smile coquettishly as he adjusts her seat belt. In one deft motion, he folds the wheelchair and lifts it onto the back of the cart, then nods to me. "We'll see you in a few minutes. Ready, Mary?"

"Ready, Chris!" she exclaims. She turns and waves, smiling like a schoolgirl who's landed next to the quarterback on a homecoming float.

I walk quickly to our room. It's not until I'm on my way back that I look around at the landscape—really look, for the first time since we arrived. The fog that covered the mountains last night and this morning is lifting now, but a few wisps of bluish haze remain. The elevation of this place has a disorienting effect. It's as though I'm not *on* a mountain but, rather, floating above the range. Even wearing my guitar on my back and crossing the cumbersome gravel, I feel light and airy. Free.

The golf cart is just up ahead. My mother is situated in her wheelchair again, and Chris leans toward her from the driver's seat, chatting amiably. They don't notice me until I'm almost upon them.

"Well, Mary, I see my services are no longer needed," says Chris. "I'll be back later to take you to lunch."

"I can't thank you enough," my mother trills. "See you soon!"

"Having fun?" I ask as Chris whirs off in his cart.

"Oh my," she replies. "I certainly am. Chris is rather easy on the eyes, don't you think?"

I laugh. "I have to hand it to you, Mom. You've still got it."

She slaps my hand lightly in protest, but giggles along with me as I push her chair up the ramp. Inside is a large classroom with one wall entirely lined with windows that face the mountains, now fully lit by the sun.

"Isn't it beautiful here?" she says.

"It is," I agree.

Chairs are arranged in a circle and a few people are already here, awaiting the instructor, Paul Fitzgibbon. He's a writing professor from a local college who's published several books of poetry. The room is almost full by the time he enters, his arms laden with stacks of paper, tote bags hanging off each shoulder.

"Hello, Writers of Planet Earth!" he booms. "I come bearing gifts!"

He bustles around the room, handing out stapled packets and reaching into his bags to present each of us with a single bell, the kind you might find sewn to the toe of a Christmas stocking. We look at each other, bemused, and by the time he finally takes a seat in the circle, Paul Fitzgibbon has our full attention.

"Welcome to The Music of Writing," he says. "We have just ninety minutes together today, and so much to do." He glances down at his bags with a worried expression. I'm so curious about the bell in my hand that I find myself sharing his concern. If the bags hold similarly intriguing items, how indeed will we get through it all?

"Let's start with this." With the flourish of a magician, he reaches out one arm and opens his hand to reveal the jingle bell at rest in the center of his palm, then closes his fingers around it. "Please hold your bell as I'm holding mine," he says, "tightly in a closed fist. Really squeeze it." He looks around the room to make sure our knuckles are sufficiently white. He nods approvingly.

"Now shake your fist," he instructs, and he demonstrates with gusto, violently moving his entire forearm as if the bell in his grasp has committed a terrible crime. We all follow suit.

"Can you hear anything?" he asks. We shake our heads along with our shaking fists. I glance over at my mother. The tempo of her movements is half the speed of the rest of the group's, and jerkier, but I can tell that she's shaking with all her might, that she's losing herself in the joy of her own physicality.

"Now stop," says Paul. We do. "Loosen your grip around the bell. Hold it very lightly. And now let's shake again."

The room is alive with the tinkling sound of bells. Everyone looks at one another in wonder at this discovery: bells can ring! My mother's face lights up with her delight. We sound the bells until, with a grand gesture, Paul signals for us to stop.

"When it comes to writing, and also in life," he says, moving his gaze around the circle so that we understand he is speaking directly to each of us, "we sometimes hold on too tightly. In writing, we try to force the words to do our bidding. And in life, we try to force the world to give us what we desire. I would like you to keep these bells as a reminder to loosen your grip, to let the music of language and life *play*."

The ninety minutes seem to hold the wisdom of ninety years. We receive more "gifts" from Paul's grab bags—little rubber ducks encourage us to ride the waves of life; plastic coins remind us to mine our pain for writing "gold"—and we respond to several prompts. I take my guitar out onto a porch lined with Adirondack rocking chairs, where I look out at the mountains, palm my bell, and let fresh lyrics pour onto the page. When the session ends, I feel as though I'm coming out of a trance. My mother looks dazed as well. I reach to put my guitar back in its case as a striking woman I'd noticed in the group approaches. She's in her sixties, with dyed black hair, a denim dress, and a turquoise-studded belt.

"What kind of music do you play?" she asks, nodding toward my guitar.

Most of the people here seem friendly to a fault, but this lady's expression is steely. Intimidating. Even after ninety minutes under Paul's spell.

"Oh, I haven't been playing long," I say, feeling embarrassed. "I'm not very good."

"She's being modest," my mother interjects. "She has a lovely singing voice."

I shake my head in protest, and the woman waves a dismissive hand. "If you know three chords and can hold a tune, you're good enough for me. Bring your guitar to the main hall after dinner. A few of us who brought instruments are getting together to jam."

I glance at my mother, and she bobs her head in encouragement. "Thanks," I sputter. "I'll be there."

"Great," says the woman coolly.

After she's left the room, another woman, heavyset and wearing a chunky sweater, comes up and stage-whispers, "She used to be kind of famous, you know. She and her husband put out a few albums in Nashville. I heard she's even played with Bob Dylan!"

"Oh God," I say, the color draining from my face. If the standard is knowing three chords and holding a tune, I'll be okay. But hanging with Dylan's set is something else entirely.

"Don't worry. She doesn't seem like it at first, but she's the nicest lady. She comes to this retreat every year." She pats my hand reassuringly and waddles off.

My mother is looking at me, wide-eyed. "Molly, my darling," she says. "This is the most excitement I've had in a long time."

I laugh. "Well, I'm glad of that. Now let's get you to your chariot. We don't want to keep Chris waiting."

As I push her wheelchair out the door and into the magnificent sunshine, I realize: my migraine is gone.

THAT EVENING AFTER DINNER, I strap on my guitar and push my mother's chair to the musicians' gathering place. I'm trying to fight off impostor syndrome, which threatens to send me running in the other direction.

The steely woman—whose name, I've learned, is Lorraine—has one foot on the hearth of the unlit fireplace as she tunes her fiddle. An older man sits to one side with an acoustic guitar, and a younger woman stands nearby with a ukulele. I have never "jammed" with strangers in my life. But what's most daunting is the small crowd that has gathered. Perhaps thirty people are spread out around the room, looking toward us expectantly. Among them is the heavyset woman who told me of Lorraine's fame. She gives me an encouraging smile.

When we've finished tuning, Lorraine says to the man with the guitar, "So what shall we play?"

"Don't look at me!" he says.

"And I'm terrible at remembering lyrics," says the woman with the ukulele. She nods to me. "What songs do *you* know?"

"Ummm . . . ," I stammer. "I know 'Sound of Silence.' But my voice is kind of low. I can't do the melody. Mom, can you be Garfunkel? You know the lyrics."

"Oh my," says my mother, blushing. "My voice isn't very strong these days."

"We'll help you, Mary!" shouts someone from the crowd. I've noticed that everyone at the retreat seems to know my mother's name.

"Great. What key?" asks Lorraine, looking at me.

I gulp. "I'm not really sure," I admit.

"Play your first chord and I'll figure it out," she says.

I put my capo on the second fret and strum.

"E minor," she says. "Everybody got it? Let's do a four-bar intro. Get us started, Tommy."

The seated guitar player taps his foot a few times and then begins with a delicate fingerpicking. The other musicians join in. I am delighted to find that I'm one of them. *I am a musician.* I nod toward my mother as I open my mouth to sing the opening lyric in the lower register. Her soprano is faint but right on pitch. Other voices in the room join hers, and the fiddle supports me in the harmony.

> *Hello darkness, my old friend,*
> *I've come to talk with you again*

At the end of the song, a hush descends over the fiddle's last mournful note, and the room erupts in cheers and applause.

I look at my mother. She is glowing.

THAT NIGHT, LYING IN our twin beds, we are both unable to sleep, too keyed up from the marvels of the day.

"Molly," she says, "I want to thank you again for bringing me here."

"It's okay, Mom. You don't have to thank me. I'm having a great time, too." I mean this. Something has shifted inside me today. For starters, I haven't thought about Karl at all. Not once, except now, to note that he no longer consumes my mind.

"I'm so glad, honey. And I'm so glad your headache is gone."

"You and me both."

We lie in silence for a moment, and then she continues, her voice breaking: "I never could have done this on my own. But even if I could have, I never *would* have done this on my own."

"What do you mean?" I ask, propping myself on one elbow to face her. Once she is settled in bed—her body correctly positioned on the absorbent pad, an extra pillow under her knees—she tries not to move too much, lest we need to repeat the arduous process of getting her situated.

"I really admire your courage," she says. "Signing up for a retreat. Renting a car and driving in the mountains. Playing guitar for a crowd. You do things that I never could."

Her words settle over me and I take them in, examining them for truth. "Thank you, Mom. I don't always feel so courageous." I want to ask her something, but I don't know how. She senses the question in the air and remains quiet. "Do you remember when you first started getting your Parkinson's symptoms? How you wondered if it was because of your 'repressed rage'?"

"Did I say that?" she asks, sounding genuinely surprised.

Somehow, it makes sense that she's forgotten. Repression isn't undone in a day.

"Yup," I say. "You did."

"Huh," she says, taking my word for it. "Well, I've always had trouble showing anger. It has to go *somewhere,* doesn't it?"

"Yeah, it does," I agree. Lately I've been considering this idea more and more. Just as stuffing your belly can cause a stomachache, stuffing down your anger can cause all sorts of bodily pain.

My own body has shown me this truth time and time again, with increasing clarity.

My questions for my mother suddenly become clear, too. They spill out of me like water. "But I want to know where your anger came from. Because I'm trying to figure this out for myself. Was it Dad? Was it being a mom? Was it Jesus Christ and Buddha? And did having an open marriage make you feel *less* angry or *more* angry?"

She sighs, and I wait. I wait for my mother to transmit the wisdom she *must* have accrued over the course of a lifetime.

"The truth is," she says, "I really don't know."

I sink down on the bed, but it's not disappointment I feel. It's more like resignation. After all, this is the answer I expected.

"But I do know this," she continues. "And it's the most important lesson I've ever learned."

Hope and curiosity rear up in me. Maybe she does have some wisdom to impart.

"What is it?"

"Everything that happens in life," she begins, "is an opportunity to learn about yourself. Marriage. Motherhood. Relationships. Even anger and illness. Nothing that happens is good or bad in and of itself. It's all just an opportunity to learn and grow."

My skin starts to tingle, and I nod solemnly in the darkness. This moment feels almost holy.

"Mom, can I tell you something?"

"Of course, sweetie."

The story of the past few months tumbles out: what happened with Karl and Martina, my fears of Stewart loving Kiwi. I lay bare my feelings of loss and pain and sadness and confusion, and my mother listens. When I'm done, she speaks.

"Oh, sweetie, that's a lot," she says. "I'm sorry it's been hard.

But remember: everything is an opportunity to learn. *Don't waste this opportunity.*"

"Thanks, Mom," I say. "I'll try not to."

"And anyway," she adds, her tone light, as if she is dropping a balloon rather than a bomb, "my threesome wasn't *nearly* as exciting."

PART THREE

CHAPTER 14

"SO I THINK I'M ready to date again," I say to Mitchell as soon as I sit down. In lieu of couples therapy, I'm back to weekly solo sessions. Mitchell supported this change in focus. *Working on yourself will only help your marriage,* he told me. "I think I have the bandwidth for it now."

Mitchell nods. "You very well may, but let's talk about it. What's changed since your relationship with Karl ended?"

I stop to think. So much feels different.

For one, I've gotten more serious about music. I've formed a duo with a friend from guitar school, Susan, and we rehearse at least once a week, writing songs, working out vocal harmonies, and drinking wine. Having this outlet—and a new creative partnership—feeds a part of me I didn't know was starving.

And then there's boxing. I've been going to class three times a week. The gym is in an unventilated basement on the eastern edge of Chelsea. This, combined with the cockroaches in the shower, gives it a street cred that appeals to me. The other women in class have cool nicknames—Sparky, Texas, Storm. I'm still called Molly, but when I warm up with Storm, trading jabs and hooks, I feel tough, a new strength and confidence in my body.

"It's a bunch of things," I say to Mitchell. "It's guitar and boxing, and new friendships. I feel like I'm taking care of parts of myself I've neglected since the kids were born. And none of it is about pleasing others. It's all for me."

Suddenly, I know the real answer to Mitchell's question. I know what's different. *Maybe I fixed the hole in my bucket,* I almost say, but I don't want to jinx myself.

I DECIDE TO WAIT a bit longer before going back on OkCupid. Stew and I are planning a trip to Maine while the kids are at camp, and I don't want to be distracted. The idea of being alone with each other for a whole week is exciting, but a needle of anxiety pokes at me, a self-imposed pressure to prove that my bucket no longer leaks, that I don't need Stewart to fill me up, to "make" me happy.

Of course, the intention to not put pressure on myself leads me to do just that. So when we check into the Bar Harbor Inn and Stew lies on the bed, busying himself with his phone, I feel myself reeling into familiar territory. Before I can put words to my thoughts, I flop next to Stewart, facedown, in a dramatic pose of despair.

"Already?" he exclaims. "I'd ask if it's something I said, but I haven't said a word."

"I know!" I moan. "I'm ruining our vacation and it hasn't even started."

"Baby. You have plenty of time to ruin our vacation later. Let's just talk for now. What's going on?"

I laugh. "I guess I'm afraid I'm *going* to ruin it."

"Would you like *me* to ruin it first and get it over with?"

I laugh again. But he's not far from the truth. "I'm kind of afraid of that, too. As soon as I saw you grab your phone, I assumed it was Kiwi or some other woman, and I'm worried you're going to text your girlfriends all week and you and I won't use this time to reconnect."

He turns his phone toward me to display a game of solitaire. "Not texting," he says. "I doubt Kiwi will text much anyway. She's working a lot these days."

"But she's not the only one who writes you. Maybe just turn off your notifications?"

He goes into his settings, then puts his phone on the bedside table. "Done. And now I have a wife I need to ravage."

OVER THE NEXT THIRTY-SIX hours, we have sex (*twice!*), eat all the lobster-based foods we can find (lobster salad, lobster omelets, lobster-stuffed lobster tails), and pass a few rainy hours playing Crazy Eights and chess at a café. On the morning of our second full day, the sun is shining as we drive to Acadia National Park for a hike. I've limited myself to one cup of coffee so I won't have to pee on the trail, but it's not nearly enough to stave off a caffeine-withdrawal headache. We park at the trailhead, and Stew looks at the map while I put on sunscreen. When I'm done, I hand it to him.

"Can you put this in the backpack?"

"Really?" He looks at the value-size bottle. "Why do you need so much shit for a four-hour hike?"

"Four hours? But we didn't pack a lunch! I thought we were doing a short one today."

"Molly, I don't want to go on a flat trail that's filled with kids and dogs. Aren't we here to explore Acadia?"

"I know, and it'll be fun," I say glumly. "Let me just grab a couple of granola bars from the glove compartment."

Once he packs my snacks—and removes my water and ChapStick for one last sip and application, then puts those back as well—we set off. Stewart hikes briskly, and I watch his strong, freckled calves bulge above the special hiking socks he bought for this occasion. I feel like I'm running to keep up, and this annoys me. After a few minutes, I shout louder than necessary, "Can you wait for me, please?"

Stew sighs and turns around. "You do realize that if we go at a slower pace, it's gonna take even longer to do this loop."

"But my legs are shorter than yours," I whine. "And I didn't drink enough coffee. I have a headache."

"Okay," Stew says, bowing his head in defeat. "Why don't you go ahead of me and set the pace."

"Can I have some water first?"

His head drops lower, and he retrieves one of my three water bottles from his pack.

We walk in silence for a while, and I start to feel better. The air is easily twenty degrees cooler than in Brooklyn, and I can almost feel my blood being oxygenated by the glorious trees surrounding us. I concentrate on aligning my breath with my step as birdsong fills my ears.

"It really is beautiful here," I say over my shoulder. "How did you pick this trail?"

"Kiwi came here last year. She and Evan take the kids hiking all the time. She said it's a good warm-up to do on day one."

My headache flares for a moment as I digest these details.

"Her *kids* did this trail?" I say, looking at the steep path ahead. "Isn't the youngest, like, five years old?"

"Yeah," he says, laughing. "They're a pretty outdoorsy family. It must be those New Zealand genes."

"I guess so," I say, forcing a laugh as well. Why does this information bother me so much? Maybe it makes me feel like a terrible mother. I'm raising my kids in a concrete jungle and I let them play video games for hours on end. On top of this, I'm angry at myself. How has my jealousy managed to barge in on this moment of union with nature's majesty? What the fuck happened to my fixed bucket? As I wrestle with myself, Stewart mistakes my silence for an invitation to keep talking.

"Did I ever tell you about the time Kiwi punched Evan in the face?" he asks, still laughing to himself. My body tenses, but I don't speak. "It was a few years ago, back when they first opened their marriage. Kiwi had a bunch of dates before Evan found anyone he liked. So he finally goes on a date with another woman—with Kiwi's full blessing—and as soon as he gets back home, she punches him. With a closed fist. She almost broke his nose."

I stop so suddenly that Stewart steps on the back of my shoe. I turn around, tempted to punch him in the face as well.

"Why the hell are you telling me this?" I spit. "Why is Kiwi's anger so goddamn amusing, and *my* anger is something I'm never supposed to talk about?"

I watch Stewart's face change from surprise to something else. Like he's just solved a puzzle he's been working on for years. His body goes slack.

"We talk about your anger all the time, Molly," he says. "In fact, I can't remember the last time we had a conversation where you weren't angry or I wasn't worried that I'd *make* you angry. And the second I let my guard down—" He cuts himself off and starts marching ahead of me up the trail. The leaves and twigs under his feet pop and snap like firecrackers.

"So that's it?" I shout after him. "We're done talking? And you're going to just leave me alone in the woods?"

"Yes! I'm fucking done!" he shouts, but he stops walking and leans against a tree trunk. When he speaks again, he drops each word like a heavy burden: "I think you *want* to be angry at me. Every conversation with you is a minefield. It's like you're waiting for me to step into some taboo topic—except I never know what's going to trigger the explosion. I'm exhausted, Molly. I can't do this anymore."

"So you want to close the marriage?" I say, setting my next trap.

"You *know* that's not what I want," he says. I silently celebrate this victory. "And maybe it's what you want today. But admit it: if Karl were still in the picture, we wouldn't be having this discussion. And if you meet someone new tomorrow, we won't be having it then, either."

I examine a mushroom growing out of a dead branch to divert my attention from the truth of his words.

"You know what's ironic?" he says. It seems like he's talking to himself, so I don't bother answering. But I look up from the mushroom. "Kiwi thinks you're amazing. The story I just told you about how she punched Evan? She told me that when we were discussing *you*. I told her how you're taking a break from dating, but you're still letting *me* date—which is amazing, Molly. I don't take it for granted. And Kiwi was saying how much she admires you for being able to do that—for giving me something that makes me happy, even though it's hard for you. And I do thank you for that. I really do."

I look back down at the mushroom as I turn this over in my mind. I did give Stew an ultimatum about couples counseling, but I've never demanded that we close the marriage. I fantasized about it with Mitchell in therapy a few times, but I always came back to the same thing: I know Stewart is happier this way. And I also know, deep down, that it's good for me, too, whether I'm dating other people or not. I'm learning to be responsible for my own happiness. I visualize my bucket for a moment and mentally patch over the leak that has sprung from the bottom.

"You're welcome," I say. "Sorry about the land mines."

"It's okay," he says. "But are there any more up ahead?" He motions toward the trail.

"I wish I knew," I answer. He hoists the pack onto his back and gestures for me to take the lead again. "Just one more thing. Promise you won't get mad?"

"I won't get mad," he says, looking wary.

"Can you get out my water bottle?"

He groans, taking off the pack again. "You're a real pain in the ass, you know that?"

"Takes one to know one," I say.

THE LAST DAY OF our trip falls on our seventeenth anniversary. We never do gifts—just cards. A few months ago, when thoughts of Karl still haunted me, I opened one of my dresser drawers, and there, lying atop a mass of sweatpants, was an old one from Stewart:

SOMEDAY YOU WILL FIND THIS CARD IN A DRAWER

It was the third time I'd indeed found the card in a drawer. Each time, I put it back in the narrowest drawer at the top of the dresser, and each time, it slipped down through the empty space behind the runners, landing somewhere new. My top drawer is stuffed with cards Stew has given me over the years, but this is the only one that ever relocates. On this occasion, it had dropped four drawers down and positioned itself front and center. I knew what was printed on the inside, but I still felt a flutter of anticipation as I opened it.

SOMEDAY YOU WILL FIND THIS CARD IN A DRAWER
AND WE WILL STILL BE IN LOVE.

Then, in Stewart's meticulous hand, were two pages of beautiful, hilarious prose. I once caught Stewart at his laptop composing a card for me. I hadn't realized he always typed up a draft before copying it over with a pen.

This year, I've tried extra hard to write a card to Stew that approaches the high bar he's set. But as usual, my card to him is nothing compared to the one he gives me. The front cover of his shows a woman bending at the waist, hands under her feet, a blissful smile on her face.

LIFE IS A LOT LIKE YOGA.

RELAX, BE FLEXIBLE . . .

I open it:

. . . AND TRY NOT TO FART.

My Beautiful Wife—

Every year I face the same decision: what kind of anniversary card best exemplifies the past year?

A sentimental one? A goofy one? Yet another "Happy Quinceañera" card? No—this year's classy choice is all about how fun this past year has been—and how good you look in yoga pants.

This card shows how we've both learned to be more accepting of each other's limitations. How marriage is a hard, sometimes challenging, struggle that leaves us both feeling happy, better, and more strongly connected. And sweatier.

And, possibly, because the only other remotely interesting card choice at CVS at 2 a.m. was "Happy Anniversary from the Dog."

I'm definitely not saying this past year has been all flowers and unicorns. I know we've had a tough time with dating stuff. Open stuff. Migraines. Holy shit. I think I bought the wrong card. This year has been a fucking mess.

But there's nobody—and I mean NOBODY—in this whole world that I'd want to face all these things with more than you. You are my wife. My friend. My therapist. The angel/devil on my shoulder. My co-pilot. My pilot. My fashion adviser.

But mostly, you're my favorite person. Ever. It's just an added bonus that you grow more beautiful and sexy with each passing year.

And you look fucking amazing in yoga pants. Worth mentioning twice.

I love you. Every sexy, sweet, quirky, kissable inch of you.

—Stew xxoo

WHEN WE RETURN TO Brooklyn, I dive back into a routine that includes work, guitar, helping Nate with his math homework, and its antidote: boxing. As I ride the F train to 23rd Street, going against the grain of commuters on their way home from midtown offices, I like the way my boxing bag fills the space between my feet. I like rummaging through the bag to find my extra-large water bottle. The heft of my gloves. The smooth purple hand wraps, the rolling of which is my new favorite laundry ritual.

At 14th Street, I feel my phone buzz. I keep forgetting that some subway stations have Wi-Fi now. Sighing, I pull it out of the zipped side pocket. Soon there won't be any place on earth where I can ignore emails and texts.

It's a notification from OkCupid. I'm back on the app with a new mindset. For my profile pic, I've chosen a photograph of myself onstage at an open mic—playing guitar, singing, and looking fierce. I want to present myself as a woman who's strong, who has her own passions and doesn't need to borrow anyone else's. In the photo, I'm singing a blues song I wrote right after Karl ghosted me, while Stew was out on a date with Kiwi:

You come home every night to your favorite lie
You come home every night to your favorite lie
Don't worry 'bout me, baby, I'm just fine

But now I really *am* fine. Most of the time, anyway. Mitchell has assured me that the occasional leak in my bucket doesn't mean all progress is lost. It's true that I'm able to patch up holes more quickly than before. And I'm determined to heed my mother's advice, to use dating as an opportunity to learn about myself and grow.

I shoulder my bag and ascend the stairs at 23rd Street. Once I'm out in the open air, I scroll through a barrage of messages. The most recent one is from a guy who also messaged me yesterday. And the day before. There's a close-up of his face, unsmiling but scruffy in a cute way. He has a full head of dark hair, thick lips, and light blue bedroomy eyes, direct and pleading.

Name: Scott
Age: 43
Height: 5'8"
Body Type: Average
Relationship Status: Ethically Non-monogamous (married)

A little short, but my age! And in an open marriage! I scan the messages. The first one is a standard intro:

Hi, Molly. I'm Scott, and I'm new to this whole open marriage thing. I also have two kids and love music. I look forward to hearing from you!

The second message was sent yesterday:

Hi again, Molly. Scott here. Sorry to bother you. I'm sure you have much better things to do. But my wife has gotten like 4,000 replies to her profile already, and I have zero! You seem to have your shit together in the ways of ENM, and I'd really appreciate your help. What am I doing wrong? Is it because I live in New Jersey? Thanks so much for any advice you can offer.

The final message was sent five minutes ago, sparking the alert on my phone:

Molly, it's Scott. I feel like such an idiot writing you three times in a row. I think I'm just going to shut down my OKC account if I don't hear from you. No pressure or anything. I just wanted to explain in case you don't see this for weeks and then write me back and think I'm ignoring you. I promise I'm not crazy. I'm actually pretty nice. According to my friends, anyway. But they're all 25-year-old assholes, so who knows?

I shake my head, but I'm grinning. Who *is* this guy? Even if it's a ploy, the terrible execution makes it charming. I decide to write him back.

Scott!! Don't do anything rash! I've been busy but I'll take a closer look at your profile later tonight. Jersey certainly doesn't help. And you're 43, right? What's with the 25-year-old friends??

I hit Send and walk into the boxing gym. Storm and Texas wave to me and I head toward them, wrapping my hands into purple cocoons, ready to counter whatever blows may come.

CHAPTER 15

THAT SATURDAY, I MAKE plans to meet Scott at Rough Trade, a record store and music venue so cool I've never heard of it. He's going with some friends to see a punk band called Beach Slang.

This is why my friends are so much younger than I am, he explains in a text. *They're the only ones who have my taste in music.*

Since he lives in Jersey and doesn't get to Brooklyn often, I've told him I'll stop by. *But this doesn't count as a "real" date,* I write. I'm trying to be cautious, to not dive into anything too quickly.

I get it, he replies. *Plus I'm guessing Beach Slang isn't your usual jam. Haha.*

But he wants to know everything about *my* music. What do I like to listen to? What songs do I play on the guitar? What does my voice sound like? The day before we meet, I record myself playing "Blackbird" and send it to him.

Your voice made me cry, he writes.

In the taxi on the way to Rough Trade, I review my reservations about Scott. I'm loath to admit it, but the things that have me concerned are the same things that excite me most. Scott hangs with a young crowd. He used to be a drummer. Since his kids were born, his kit has been in storage, but he's played in a couple of different bands over the years. He smokes, possibly drinks too much, and hates his day job. He's a "bad boy" but appears to be a sweet one who wears his heart on his sleeve.

When I step out of the car, I see Scott standing in front of the club. His hair is dyed jet black and combed forward on his forehead. His flannel shirt is open, revealing a weathered concert T-shirt underneath. He drops his cigarette onto the sidewalk and stomps it with the heel of his boot. I feel a tingle when I see his sleepy eyes, a shade of blue that reminds me of sadness.

"Molly?" he says as he walks toward me. His voice is an octave deeper than I expected, full-throated and sexy. "Oh my God. You're so beautiful." The tingle intensifies and radiates outward. He's standing in front of me now. He might have fudged his height, as men on the shorter side often do, but he's still an inch taller than I am.

"Hi, Scott." The awed look on his face is intoxicating but makes me embarrassed just the same.

"Do you want to go somewhere? To talk?" He's already taking my hand.

"You don't want to see the show?" I ask, staring dumbly at my hand in his. To be honest, I'm relieved to not have to meet his friends, Jersey boys who I'm sure I wouldn't be able to stand, who'd make it impossible for me to suspend my disbelief about Scott. The way he looks at me already feels like a drug I need to function.

"No way. I don't want to miss a second with you." He continues to hold my hand in his and drinks me with his eyes. I'm wearing an outfit that I hope looks more Williamsburg than Park Slope: black jumpsuit, oversized belt, strappy sandals. "You're such a rock star."

The tingling twists into something less pleasurable, and I pull my hand away instinctively. What am I doing? Outsourcing my self-worth again so soon?

"No, I'm not," I say, my voice rising in something akin to anger. Scott's face falls, and he looks almost frightened. I soften. "It's just . . . you don't know me at all."

"I'm so sorry. You're right. I don't know you. But I want to. I really want to. There's a bar on the corner. Do you want to grab a drink?"

We walk along the rough, cobblestoned streets and I realize I've slipped my hand into his again. I've never dated someone so close to my height, and I note the ease with which we fall into step with each other. What exactly is happening? I'm simultaneously comfortable and off-kilter.

We find two seats at the bar, and I notice that everyone around us is under thirty, including the black-clad, heavily tattooed bartenders. I feel silly ordering a glass of wine, but I do.

"Make it two," says Scott in his baritone. He turns to me and leans in. "You're already making me more sophisticated."

I laugh and reach for my wallet, but he waves me off. I watch him sort through the debris in his pocket—an almost-empty pack of cigarettes, two lighters, an incongruous ChapStick—to find a wad of cash. He peels off a twenty and a five and turns back to face me.

"Okay, Beautiful. Tell me everything about yourself."

He gazes at me in rapt attention as I go through my curated repertoire of stories: growing up with my wild sister, joining and quitting my mother's cult, teaching English in Costa Rica.

Scott asks lots of follow-up questions and dodges my attempts to get him to talk. But I pick up a few tidbits. His mother had been a stewardess. His father used to be a cop in upstate New York, but ran over his foot with a lawn mower, severing his toe, and had to take a desk job with a precinct in Florida. Scott spent seven years in college before finally graduating. He works in purchasing—in a series of temp positions, really, which ensures that he never has to take a job too seriously, that he can go to shows in the city on weeknights and work hungover, functioning well enough on five hours of sleep. He has a daughter and a son. His wife, Diana, works in the hotel industry; open marriage was her idea. He hadn't been into it. Until meeting me, that is.

"You don't want to hear about my life. I'm boring," Scott tells me. "But I could sit here all night and listen to your stories."

THREE DAYS LATER, SCOTT and I go out again. *This date counts,* he texts. He takes the bus into Port Authority and asks me to meet him at a bar in the East Village.

The Ramones used to hang out there, he writes. *It's an iconic place. My friend's band wrote a song about it.* He sends me a link, and I listen on the train on my way to Second Avenue. It's got a poppy punk sound, and the lyrics are surprisingly intelligible.

> *I have heard some places can change how you feel*
> *It's not something you can see but I think that it's real*

I think that it's real, too. When I walk through the nondescript door, I *do* feel different. There are Christmas lights around the horseshoe-shaped bar. Green leather seats. Wood-paneled walls. A deep cut by an '80s band I recognize but can't name coming out of the speakers. This place makes me feel not *in* my element, exactly, but in an element I'd like to occupy. Why did I get so angry when Scott called me a rock star? It's clearly what I want to be. Perhaps it's even what I am. I'm wearing a denim miniskirt tonight, an item that's been hanging in my closet for years, waiting for my legs to look like they did at age twenty-eight. But I no longer care about the knee wrinkles that arrived with Daniel's birth. Boxing has added muscle to my calves, and as I watch my mother struggle to walk, I value my own body's strength. Plus, I *like* being forty-three. I wouldn't go back in time for anything. Confidence is what makes a rock star, right?

Scott is sitting on a couch in the corner. When he sees me, he stands and smiles in his sad, sleepy way.

"Hey there, Beautiful," he says. His deep voice soothes me, like the chanting of Tibetan monks.

We hug and I take in his smell, cigarettes and soap and the buttery sweetness of rum. I sit down next to him, and my hand finds his. We spend the next two hours sipping cocktails with little umbrellas, snacking on fries and kimchi tacos, talking about music, commenting on the eccentric regulars scattered around the bar. What is it about this guy? In so many ways, we're nothing alike. Yet there's a familiarity between us, like I've known him forever—or, more importantly, like he's known me. And then it hits me.

This is how I felt on my first date with Stewart.

STEW AND I MET in Manhattan, at Nina's birthday party. I was with William, before we broke up and I moved to the city to live with Nina. Tall, athletic, and intellectual, William was the man I thought I'd marry. He was also Stewart's opposite.

Stew was decidedly not my type. He fit every negative stereotype of a Long Island Jew. He was loud, brash, and wore pants with pleats. His jokes were either offensive or self-deprecating. I found him obnoxious. But a few months later, when Stew learned that my relationship with William was over, he pestered Nina for information, wanting to know if I would go out with him. He liked me. And I needed to be liked. I needed it desperately. I agreed to give him a chance.

On our first date, Stewart took me to impressive places: a bar with cushy armchairs and a fireplace, a Thai restaurant with vertically arranged food. During that evening together, Real Stew peeked out from his hiding place behind Performer Stew, whom I had met at the party. And I liked Real Stew. I liked him a lot. Real Stew made me laugh. He asked good questions, he listened, and he laughed at my jokes, too. We went back to his apartment, and

I shocked us both by getting naked. Unlike the staid, missionary-position sex I'd been having with William for four years, sex with Stewart was messy and noisy and *fun*.

After a few months of dating, I was on the phone with my mother, gushing about this new guy. That's when she asked me her most vital question: *How do you feel about yourself when you're with him?*

Stewart made me feel interesting. Funny. Sexy. I told my mother that no matter what happened with Stew, I would never settle for less. But I *had* settled. Since opening our marriage, I'd dated so many men who made me feel like not quite enough. Objectified. Unvalued.

Until now.

"I WANT YOU TO sing for me," says Scott. How does he know that this is the way to my heart?

"Okay," I say, blushing as I get an idea. "I know a place we can go."

"Wait," he says. "Can I do something first?"

He puts his hand on my face, holding me in the steadiness of his gaze. We look at each other for a long moment. And then he kisses me. His hands slide into my hair, and he tastes me, tentative but hungry, as if my mouth is a treat he wants to savor, to make last.

It's a five-minute walk to Sing Sing. It's been years—seven? eight?—since I was here with Matt, but some part of my reptilian brain recalls the yearning I felt that night. The guy at the desk directs us to room number five. I'm not sure if I feel relief or disappointment that it's not the same room Matt and I shared. Scott sits on the couch and folds his jacket like an audience member at the Met. Only the Marlboro Lights poking out of his shirt pocket give him away.

"What should I sing?" I ask him.

"Whatever you want, Beautiful." His eyes stay with me as I flip through the book of song titles.

"I've been working on something by Sheryl Crow," I say. "Maybe I'll try that one."

"Whatever you want," he repeats.

I punch the number into the remote and turn on the microphone. The intro music starts, and a cheesy video of a moon rising over the ocean comes on. Scott and I both laugh, and the brand of tension in the room shifts.

I've always had trouble making eye contact when I sing, and I close my eyes for the first verse. When I open them, Scott is watching me so intently that I get out only a word or two before I need to look away. The lyrics feel like an explanation: *I have a face I cannot show, I make the rules up as I go.*

But when I get to the chorus, my gaze locks onto him before I realize what's happening.

Are you strong enough to be my man? I ask. Scott sits with his arm stretched along the back of the couch, his boot making a figure four with the opposite knee. His scruffy face begs to be touched, and his eyes don't leave mine. As I hold the last note of the song, I'm still looking right at him. I take a step forward and practically fall onto his lap. It happens quickly, naturally. Our mouths connect. His fingers reach under my skirt and slide beneath my panties. I orgasm so quickly, I wonder if this is a dream. A hammering on the door assures me that it's not.

"No sex!" shouts the voice attached to the knocking hand. "No sex allowed!"

Scott and I separate, and I follow his eyes up to a corner of the room. A video camera points down at us.

"Smile, Beautiful!" he says, laughing.

I bury my face in my hands. But I'm laughing, too.

"Oh my God, we have to leave. You go first," I say.

He grabs our stuff and takes my hand. I keep my eyes on the ground and follow him out the door. He strides down the hall, and I practically run to keep up, trying not to trip. I've had enough mortification for one night.

"Sorry about that," he says to the desk staff in his throaty voice. Despite his words, his tone is far from contrite. It's sexy as hell.

We spill onto the street, laughing and running, our hands still joined. When we get to the corner, Scott goes deadpan.

"No sex allowed!" he shouts in perfect mimicry, setting us both off into spasms again. When we catch our breath, he squeezes my hand and pulls me closer. I like the firmness of his grip. I'm practically swooning. "When can I see you again?"

"It might be a little while." I'm genuinely disappointed at my own answer, and his face mirrors my feeling. "I have a conference upstate next week."

"That sucks," he says.

"It really does," I say. "It's going to be the most boring thing in the world. But I did a Google search for open mics up there, and I found one on Thursday. So at least I have one night to look forward to."

"Can I come?" he asks, his face brightening.

I laugh, assuming he's kidding.

"I'm serious. I can take the train up after work on Thursday. I'll take a personal day Friday."

I look at him, hesitating. "I'm not allowed to have sleepovers. It's one of our rules."

"I totally get that," he says, taking a small step back and gesturing with his hands to illustrate this boundary. "But my wife works for Hyatt, remember? I can get my own room."

He looks at me with such straightforward hope that I allow myself to imagine it. Away from the kids, away from self-imposed curfews, a night full of music and possibility.

"Let me talk to Stewart about it," I say, excitement surfacing in my voice.

"Of course. And I'll talk to Diana. But I'm sure she'll be cool with it. She's dating this new guy that she can't shut up about." There's a tinge of disgust in Scott's voice as he says this. I look at him quizzically, and he hurries to add, "So she's psyched I'm into somebody, too."

I want to hear him say it again. I play coy. "You're into me, huh?"

"Molly." The way he says my name—a full sentence all by itself—makes my head feel floaty. "You have no fucking idea." As if to give me a clue, he kisses me again.

I think about this kiss on the taxi ride home. It's not only Scott's mouth that fits with mine just so. It's also how his hands cradle the back of my head. How our bodies press against each other. And something more. If a kiss were a dance, then Scott doesn't exactly lead; nor does he follow. Or maybe he leads and follows so expertly I can't tell which is which. It's as though he anticipates by a fraction of a moment where my lips, my tongue will go, and he meets me there, at a place that's unexpected and inevitable all at once.

The Q train rumbles past as my taxi crosses the Manhattan Bridge. It jolts me out of my reverie. If I'm going to talk to Stewart about meeting Scott upstate, I'd better do it soon. Maybe even tonight.

When I get home, I see Stew through the basement window, working in his studio. Darkness, like a one-way mirror, hides me from view. He leans forward, his hands on the piano keyboard, his eyes intent on the screen before him, his body in motion to the rhythm of the music pouring in through his headphones.

My husband.

I'm seeing him with new eyes. A creator. A provider. A man of passion who has built a business out of making music, the thing he loves most in this world. For so many years, I've resented Stewart's dedication to his work. Stewart's vocation was my archrival, competing with me for his attention. But now my heart swells with tenderness and appreciation for him, for who he is and what he does.

A glimmer of an idea is forming alongside this feeling. Is it possible that my being happy with another man makes me love my husband more, not less? I can't explain how this works, but the evidence is collecting inside me. I am like a crucible where magical ingredients come together to create something new.

IT'S THURSDAY, AND SCOTT texts me from his hotel, next door to mine. When I asked Stewart how he'd feel about this plan, assuring him that it wouldn't be an actual overnight because Scott was staying at a different hotel, Stew rolled his eyes.

"Seriously, Molly? Just let the poor guy sleep over!"

"Really? You wouldn't mind?"

"I mean, that rule is mostly for the kids' sake, right? If you're on a work trip, and you already have my blessing to have sex, I don't think the sleeping part is such a big deal."

"I guess so." But then an image arose in my mind of Stewart waking up next to a slumbering Kiwi, her hair covering the face I've still never seen. A sharp pang of jealousy drove me to disagree. "But sleeping together can be very intimate. I don't think I'm ready for it. Scott's wife gets free hotel rooms at the Hyatt anyway, and I have a booking at the Marriott."

"Suit yourself. But don't worry about it on my account. Just have fun."

Just have fun, I remind myself now. But I'm exhausted from two days of working the conference, and open mics always wreak havoc on my nerves. Knowing that Scott will be there makes me even jumpier.

I head down to the parking lot with my guitar strapped to my back, enjoying the intrigued looks from conference attendees hanging out in the lobby. I drive one-tenth of a mile to the front of the Hyatt and grab my phone to text Scott, but he's already standing out front, stepping on a cigarette and looking even more nervous than I feel. I roll down the window and wave.

"Hi, Beautiful," he says, smiling weakly.

"Hi, Scott," I say. He gets into the passenger seat. Stewart loves to drive. So does my father. This may be the first time since Driver's Ed that I've chauffeured a man anywhere. "Are you okay?"

"Just tired," he says, buckling his seat belt. "I didn't sleep well last night. I was excited to see you." He glances at me shyly.

I take in each detail of this scene in rapid succession. The cigarette, his anticipation, and the tenderness of his gaze release a giddiness in me. But almost against my will, my attraction is tempered by other mundane aspects: the seat belt, his slouched posture, his taciturn manner. Why is reality so unsexy?

The open mic is about twenty minutes away, along a winding road with no dividing line. A sheet of fog descends as we pass a cemetery. I'm far from home with a virtual stranger in my car.

What the hell am I doing? I wonder.

Our conversation suddenly feels stilted, and I can't muster the strength to continue it.

"Wanna see what's on the radio around here?" I say. This suggestion brings Scott to life, and he scans through the stations until he hears a song by the Clash. He tweaks the bass level, and when he's satisfied, he leans back, his body relaxed and easy again.

I pull into the parking lot of the bar, a converted barn complete

with silo and red paint. Scott opens the back door to grab my guitar, then hands it to me.

"I'd offer to carry it, but I don't want to steal your thunder."

I laugh. I appreciate how he gets it, the joy of carrying my own
guitar.

Inside, I make a beeline for the chalkboard and sign up to per-
form second while Scott finds two seats at the bar. We order nachos
and beer, and I pick at the food nervously. Dan, the first guy up—
every name on the list but mine belongs to a man—is a skilled
guitarist. His fingers scurry up and down the fretboard, and I feel
my confidence waver.

"He's got nothing on you," Scott whispers to me, reading my
mind. "His voice sucks, and he plays like a robot."

"Thanks," I whisper back, unconvinced. "Maybe I should go
outside and tune."

During the applause that follows Dan's first song, I slide out
the door with my guitar and go through the comforting motions
of adjusting each string. I strum through the opening bars of Joan
Armatrading's "Down to Zero," the song Leo suggested I learn
almost two years ago. It's my first time playing it in public, and I
now feel relieved that Scott and his attentive, encouraging eyes will
be watching me, along with all the strangers in the bar.

I hear more applause, and I know Dan is done with his set. It's
my turn.

Back inside, I take the stage. I fumble with the cable that plugs
my guitar into the amp, and my hands shake as I adjust the mic
stand. Scott steadies me with his gaze.

When I start to play, the heartbeat of the music relaxes me. I
keep my eyes closed until I have to look at my left fingers forming
the troublesome B chord. Then I face front with my eyes open
and concentrate on Scott's face. He watches me sing, carefully, as

if he's soaking in details, storing them to turn over in his mind later on.

> *Take to your bed*
> *You say there's peace in sleep*
> *But you'll dream of love instead.*

I feel seen, heard, worshipped in a way I haven't experienced since the early days with Stewart. Stew and I eventually joked about the pedestal he put me on during our first years together, and I know my falling off it drew us closer. Pedestals separate. They create imbalances. When I recalled that era with Stewart, I sometimes thought about my friend Billy, who used to throw up every time he saw his future wife. That kind of adulation has to end for anything real to develop.

But this pedestal Scott has placed me on feels so good under my feet. I like the smooth, sturdy foundation of it, the intoxicating knowledge that I am someone's ideal, someone's vision of perfection.

CHAPTER 16

A FEW MONTHS INTO dating, Scott makes me a CD. The paper inside the jewel case is labeled in an impeccable hand. Nobody owns a CD player anymore, but I've always been a sucker for ink on paper. So I keep it, even after I confess my inability to play it and Scott re-creates his gift as a Spotify playlist. The songs are by melancholy indie artists I've never heard of, with seductive titles like "Vanishing Act" and "Transatlantic Love Song." I listen to the playlist every chance I get—as I cook dinner or fold laundry, on the subway ride to the boxing gym. Each note helps me relive my nights with Scott.

He has a way of holding me that feels exactly right—somewhere between Stewart's firmness and Karl's tender touch. When I lie on my side, Scott spoons me from behind. I can feel his hardness against the soft curve of my ass. Sometimes he enters me that way. Scott says words I've asked him to say. I still like being called "good girl," but now I need something else, too. *Don't worry, Beautiful. I'm not going to hurt you. I'm just going to fuck you.* He pushes down on my back and every part of me gives way and I let him enter me completely. I want to be controlled, but only insofar as I cannot control myself. When my arms flail, I need them pinned. When I start to scream, I need to be gently shushed. What I want is to be guided through a release from my body, from my mind, from my inhibitions and fears and the very core of myself. I almost always

cry after Scott makes me orgasm. Then he holds me and we do it
again—often five or six times in one night.

When Stewart and I are in bed together, he begs to hear the
details of my sex with Scott. But it takes me a while to reveal Scott's
impressive virility.

"He must be on Viagra," Stewart says dismissively.

"Yeah, probably," I say, but only to preserve Stew's ego. I don't
think it's true. I prefer to believe that Scott's perpetual erection is
about me, that his desire for me is insatiable, all-consuming.

MOST WEEKS, I LEAD at least one teacher training in New
Jersey. Scott and I meet at a budget hotel near his new temp job in
Newark. We have sex, go to a diner a few blocks away, then back to
the hotel for more sex.

One night, over dinner, Scott asks if I've seen the new Jordan
Peele movie.

"*Get Out*? Not yet. But I really want to," I say, scraping my
plate to finish off the last bite of cheese enchilada. Besides being on
my feet all day, a pre-dinner romp has given me a huge appetite.
"Have you seen it?"

"Nah, Diana's not into it. She thinks it sounds 'disturbing.'"
He makes air quotes and scoffs.

I shrug. His digs at Diana make me mildly uncomfortable, so
I try to breeze past them. "It got great reviews."

Scott pulls out his phone. "It's playing about a mile from here.
Do you want to go?"

I do. But although Stewart and I have broken most of our original open-marriage rules, I've still never seen a movie with anyone
else. And I know Stew is dying to see this one. *I'll just offer to see it
a second time,* I rationalize.

"Yeah," I say. "Let's do it."

Scott's face lights up. He scrolls through his phone, jabbing his finger and chattering as he buys the tickets. I consider pulling out my own phone to tell Stewart my plan but instead grab our check and head to the cash register to pay.

"Okay, I got tickets for the eight-forty show," he says when I get back to the table. "We're gonna have to hurry."

Scott's car is in the parking lot of the hotel. We run back and I jump into the passenger seat. "I think this is my first time in your car," I say. Aside from a half-empty pack of cigarettes and an open can of Coke in the center console, the car is tidy.

"Yeah, I guess it is," he says, smiling at me as he turns the key.

I like the way he drives. He backs out of the parking spot without using his mirrors and steers with his left hand, palming the wheel to make turns. His right hand is therefore free to adjust the radio and caress my knee.

We duck into the theater after the previews have begun. Stew requires total silence during trailers—sometimes he hears one of his own compositions or sound design elements. But Scott is uninterested in the screen. I feel his gaze, and I turn to see him grinning at me.

"You are psyched about this movie," I whisper, laughing.

"I'm psyched to be here with *you*," he corrects me. "I don't know. It's like we're really together."

I understand what he means. Somehow, sitting next to each other in this dark theater feels more intimate than sex at the hotel. *I should have texted Stewart,* I think with a twinge of guilt. I push the thought away and hook my arm around Scott's, laying my head on his shoulder. *Just enjoy this. You can deal with Stew later. Maybe he won't even care.*

Horror is the perfect genre for a movie date. I enjoy the film almost as much as I relish my own reactions to it. I gasp. I hide my face against Scott's warm, smoky flannel. I grab his bicep with both hands. Scott's into it, too. He pets my head and rubs my back and chuckles at my antics.

We leave the theater holding hands. I launch into a half-formed analysis, barely pausing for breath.

"And the cotton in his ears was so cool! It's like he's using this symbol of slavery to escape the enslavers. Jordan Peele is a genius."

"*You're* a genius," says Scott. "I didn't notice any of that stuff. But it was a great movie."

Scott is quiet as he drives back to the hotel parking lot and pulls into the spot next to my car. He looks at me with a wistful expression and reaches for my hand. "So I guess you need to get back home?"

I glance at the clock on the dashboard. It's after eleven.

"Yeah, I probably should." My head is still buzzing from the movie. I can't wait to see it again with Stew so he can help me figure out more of the symbols. What about the deer? The camera flash?

"Thanks for going to the movies with me, Beautiful," he says, looking down with a hangdog expression and stroking my hand with his thumb.

"Are you okay?"

"Yeah. I just miss you already." He regards me with his sleepy blue eyes, and my brain melts, all thoughts of cinematic motifs and Jersey Turnpike traffic puddling in my shoes.

"I miss you, too," I say. Because suddenly I do. "I'll see you next week though, right?"

"Yeah," he says. "But it's never enough."

We're silent. I keep my hand in his and study his face in profile. He looks almost pained. It's true that I miss him when we're apart, but I also love my life. My kids, my husband, my job, my neighborhood and routines. It's dawning on me now that Scott doesn't feel the same way.

His body suddenly shudders, shaking the sadness away like a

dog leaving the water. "Oh, I almost forgot," he says. He drops my hand and reaches for his phone. "I made you another playlist. I'll share it so you can listen on your drive home."

I hear my own phone ding and see "Mix for Molly #2" added to my Spotify playlists. "Thank you!" I say, leaning over to kiss him. "That's so sweet."

"This one has eighteen songs. I'll add another song each time I make you a new one."

"You're planning on making more?"

"Of course, Beautiful. I love thinking about what music you'll like."

We say lingering good-byes and I take the long way home, through Staten Island and over the Verrazzano Bridge. I'm swept up in the poetic lyrics of Scott's song choices:

> *If you need someone*
> *To comfort you*
> *When tears fall down your face*
> *I'll do all I can . . .*

> *I feel myself slip inside*
> *As I look into your eyes . . .*

> *Take the time to show you're mine*
> *And I'll be a blue moon in the dark . . .*

Listening to the music, I feel a pleasant identity shift. I'm not a wife. I'm not a mom. I'm hardly even a grown-up.

I GET HOME AFTER midnight and see the lights on in our room. When I walk in, Stew is lying on the bed watching TV.

"Hi, baby," he says, pausing his show. "How was your date?"

"It was fun," I say. A wave of guilt hits as I remember the movie. I don't want to open with this information. "Who did you go out with again tonight?" Since I took the car and Stewart couldn't drive to Kiwi, he went out in Manhattan with someone else.

"Cara," he answers.

"Is she the psychologist?" I ask.

"Nope. The actress." Stew pulls a face. "Never date an actress."

"Noted," I say, laughing. "Did you have a good time at least?"

"I did," he answers with a sigh. "But I made the mistake of telling Kiwi where I was going."

"And let me guess. She got jealous." I know about this dramatic thread between the two of them. Kiwi has reached a point of accepting her husband's other relationships. And she is on board with *my* primacy as Stewart's wife. But the fact that Stew continues to date other women is a thorn in her side. I understand her feeling this way, and I've told Stewart as much. If Scott wanted to date other women, it would probably bother me, too. I like being the new and shiny one. But at the same time, I'm relieved that Stewart isn't capitulating to Kiwi's jealousy. After all, he never capitulated to mine. For him, having a variety of partners is the whole reason for open marriage.

"Bingo," he says. "She says she wants to know if I'm out with someone else, but when I tell her the truth, she freaks out."

"Women," I say, shaking my head in mock disgust. Stew laughs out loud. Few things are more satisfying than making my husband laugh. I don't want to ruin this moment, but I still have a confession to make. I tell him about the movie.

"Are you mad?"

Stewart shrugs. "I don't *love* it. I mean, how would you feel if there was a movie you wanted to see, but I saw it with Kiwi instead?"

I'm struck by the calmness of his reaction. Are we really going to avoid a fight? "I'd feel shitty. I'm sorry, baby."

"It's okay," he says. "As long as you'll see it again with me. And lucky for you, Kiwi hates movies."

"She does? How is that even possible?"

"I don't get it either. She prefers reading."

"Scott likes movies, but he's no good at the post-film analysis. So I'm being honest when I tell you I can't wait to see it again with you. There are *so many* things I want to discuss."

"That's your punishment, then," jokes Stew. "You can't even talk to me about it until we see it together."

"You're cruel," I say, curling up on the bed beside him.

"I know," he says. And he kisses me on top of my head.

A COUPLE OF MONTHS later, on a warm day in late April, I take the subway to an appointment with Mitchell while listening to Scott's "Mix for Molly #4"—all twenty songs in order. Once I'm settled on the couch and Mitchell asks me how everything is going, I start with the playlists. How they make me feel.

He looks up at the ceiling pensively. "So I'm wondering—does this shift in identity feel authentic? Is it a part of True Molly?"

"I've been wondering the same thing," I admit. "It's kind of like boxing. Or playing guitar. These are new things I'm exploring, but they feel right. And it's all just a little bit, I don't know—badass."

He smiles at me. "Straight-A Molly is *not* a badass."

I laugh. "Definitely not."

"You know, Molly, this reminds me again of your list of Freedoms." He leafs through his notebook, looking for the page.

I nod. "I haven't thought about the Freedoms for a while. Maybe it's because I'm feeling so much freer."

"Tell me more about that," says Mitchell, abandoning his search for the list and scribbling something on his pad.

"A lot of it has to do with the kids getting older. Daniel is fifteen now, and Nate is twelve."

"That's hard to believe."

"Tell me about it," I say. "So I'm getting enough time to do my own thing. The kids seem almost disappointed on the nights I stay home."

"Do you know what I'm noticing in all of this, Molly?" says Mitchell. I wait as he finishes jotting down a note. "Rather than getting obsessed with a relationship—or with Stewart's relationships—you're focusing on yourself. It's a significant change."

I try to see myself from Mitchell's vantage point. He senses that I have more to say and stays quiet, his pen poised above the page again. "But I still get anxious," I tell him. "I worry that things are going *too* well, that it's all going to come toppling down."

He nods and makes a note.

"For example," I say, "Scott wants to go away for the weekend with me. Like a fishing trip or something. Also, Diana—his wife—wants to meet me."

"Those are big steps," Mitchell says. "My question is whether they're steps *you* want to take as well."

"I mean, I like the excitement of new experiences. But then something might go wrong."

"Indeed," says Mitchell. He looks at me evenly, a smile behind his eyes. "That's always a risk."

I MEET DIANA AT Lucey's Lounge, the same bar where I had my first date with Karl. I chose the spot for its proximity to the Bell House, where Scott and Diana have tickets to a show. It fascinates me that only a year after being so hurt by Karl, my heart seems to have healed completely. When I walk into Lucey's, there's no hint of pain. I get there a little early and take a seat at the bar.

This meeting was Diana's idea, and I agreed in part out of curiosity. Over the past few weeks, she's sent me gifts via Scott: soaps, lotions, and, most recently, a purple rubber spatula from Williams Sonoma. I, in turn, have done nothing but stalk Diana's Facebook page—wall-to-wall selfies—and with Stewart's help, I've found her profile on OkCupid.

Don't call me a MILF! This is her opening line.

Perched on my barstool, I angle my body to get a view of the front door and see Scott and Diana framed in the window. Diana pulls his arm, urging him to come inside. Scott's eyes meet mine through the glass. He gives a sharp wave, turns on his heels, and exits the scene. A moment later, in comes Diana, giggling and gesticulating broadly.

"Oh my God—he's such a pussy!" she yells, sliding one hand through pin-straight dark hair and walking toward me on two-inch heels. "He's scared to be with us together."

Diana is prettier in person than in her pictures. I expected her coiffed, put-together look, but there is something magnetic about her, too. When I hear her sultry voice, I remember that she was a DJ at a classic rock station when she and Scott met. She's wearing a low-cut T-shirt under a fitted camouflage jacket, accentuating her MILFy body. Her hair has a gloss that doesn't appear to be bottled. But the thing that strikes me most are her eyes—an otherworldly blue—which dart around so I can never quite meet them.

Talking to Diana is easy. She talks nonstop, so I rarely have to think of anything to say. Mostly, she tells me about her boyfriend, Rick. "He technically lives in Malibu, but he's pretty much bicoastal. I don't know why the fuck *anyone* would live on the East Coast if they could be in California. Have you ever been to Malibu?"

"No, I haven't. What's it like?" I say, though she doesn't need a prompt.

"So gorgeous." She takes out her phone and shows me pictures I've already seen on Facebook. "Here we are at the beach."

She continues her monologue. It sounds like the sped-up playback of a recording. I nod and coo at her photos, but my synapses are firing in another direction. There is something unsettling about her near obsession with Rick. According to Diana, he's also in an open marriage, yet they're traveling across the country to spend every other weekend together. And I now believe what Scott has told me: Diana literally can't stop talking about her boyfriend. What does this mean for their marriage? But then I remember how I behaved with Matt, with Karl. They're new to this, I tell myself. This is probably just a good old-fashioned case of new relationship energy.

Suddenly, Diana stops talking and puts down her phone. She rests her hand on top of mine, and I note the stark contrast between her perfectly manicured fingers and my short-nailed ones, complete with hard-earned calluses from playing guitar.

"Molly," she says. Her blue eyes finally meet mine. She really is beautiful. "I want you to know something. I haven't seen Scott this happy in years. You bring out the best in him."

"That's so sweet of you to say, Diana," I sputter. Is this how I've earned lotions and a rubber spatula?

"Scott told me you're going on a fishing trip together. Is that true?"

"I mean, I'm not sure," I say, rushing my words. "I haven't talked to my husband about it. And of course I'll only go if it's okay with *you*."

She throws back her head and laughs loudly. People turn to stare. Her dark hair shimmers, and her teeth glow white against her skin, tanned by the Malibu sun. "It's more than okay!" she shouts. "It's *amazing!* God knows *I'm* not going fucking fishing."

I laugh with her at the thought of those fingernails around a fishing pole, the high heels sinking into a muddy riverbank.

She glances at her watch. It looks expensive, and I wonder if it's a present from Rick. According to Scott, he's loaded and funds all of Diana's westward travel. "I gotta run. I told Scott I'd meet him at door time. You know how crazy he gets." I don't know at all, but I fake it and nod. "We gotta do something first, though. Come here for a sec."

She puts one arm around me and holds her phone in the other at a practiced angle, taking several selfies of the two of us. "I told Rick I'd send him a picture." She gathers up her things and hugs me with what feels like genuine affection before strutting out the door.

LATER THAT NIGHT, DIANA tags me on Facebook. From my perch on the toilet, I show Stew the photo as he's on his way to the shower. "Isn't she stunning?"

"Not nearly as pretty as you, baby." Stew knows exactly how to stroke my ego. He steps under the water. "And anyway, she's a type I steer clear of."

"What do you mean?"

"How do I put this delicately? She looks like a handful."

"Yeah, I get the sense she's high-maintenance." Over the sound of the water, I tell him about our conversation, about her relationship with Rick. Stew and I never bothered putting up a shower curtain in our bathroom, and I love talking to him this way, the intimacy of mundane nudity.

"That's kind of weird," Stew says, making a face. "Do you think she wants a divorce?"

He's voicing my fear. If they get divorced, where will that leave me? I retreat to the parts of my conversation with Diana that work to allay this concern.

"I don't think so," I say. "She thanked me for making Scott

happy, and why would she care about his happiness if she doesn't still love him? Plus, they have kids."

Stew reaches for a towel and rubs his head vigorously. I'm not sure if he's convinced. "Anyway, it sounds like it went well. That's great, baby."

"Thanks," I say. This is a perfect segue to talk about the possibility of my meeting Kiwi, but now doesn't seem like the right time. I'm not sure if I'm ready yet. And I have another request that takes precedence.

"What?" Stew asks, his face emerging from behind the towel with a pointed expression.

"How did you know I have something else to talk about?"

"Molly, no offense. But you *always* have something else to talk about. What is it?" He wraps the towel around his waist and reaches for his toothbrush. I let another trickle of pee escape. Since having kids, emptying my bladder always takes several attempts.

"Diana wants me to go on a trip with Scott," I ask. I know I'm being dishonest, presenting the idea as hers. "He really loves fishing, and she hates it, so she asked me to go with him instead."

Stew laughs. "Maybe Diana and I would get along after all. Fishing sucks."

"I think it sounds kind of fun," I say.

"Then you should go, baby."

"Are you sure? This is more than a sleepover. It would be a couple of nights."

"It's fine," he says. I watch him in the mirror as he squeezes the toothpaste. "Actually, Kiwi's been asking me about taking a trip, too."

"What?" I say, my body stiffening as I sit upright on the toilet. "Where?"

"Well, I told her you weren't coming with me to Vegas this year. And she asked if maybe she could go instead." Every year,

Stewart takes a work trip to Las Vegas. When we were engaged and first married, I accompanied him. The ritual was interrupted by the arrival of Daniel and Nate; then we resumed the tradition. After our trip the previous year, though, I mentioned feeling done with the Vegas scene. I always lost money, I always ate too much, and it was too hot to ever go outside. But even if *I* don't want to go to Vegas, I don't want *Kiwi* going instead.

"When were you planning on mentioning this to me?" My words feel hot as they leave my mouth.

"I wasn't going to mention it at all," he says. His tone is that of a parent explaining the art of taking turns to a cranky toddler. This fans the flames of my anger. *How dare he behave as if I'm overreacting?* "I told her you and I don't allow overnights yet, and I wanted to wait until you were comfortable with the idea. Now you're saying you want to take a fishing trip with Scott, so silly me. I assumed you were ready." He throws up his hands, and a glob of toothpaste hits the mirror. "But I see now that it's a one-way street, and if I even *talk* about going away with Kiwi, I'm some kind of insensitive monster."

I wait for him to turn out the lights in the bedroom before I leave the bathroom. We agreed long ago that *Never go to bed angry* is a stupid rule—we just ended up exhausted in the morning. And there are times when I'd much rather let my feelings percolate and settle before I give them voice.

My logical mind hears what Stewart is saying, even agrees with him. So why won't my heart listen? I think back to a piece of *Ethical Slut* wisdom I've committed to memory: "Jealousy is often the mask worn by the most difficult inner conflict you have going on right now."

It's the same conflict as always, I suppose. Myself versus my bucket.

CHAPTER 17

IN JULY, SCOTT BOOKS a cottage near a fishing reservoir in Mount Kisco. Stewart wants the car for the weekend and offers to drop me off at Scott's house.

"I'd like to meet him," he says. The thought of this is both thrilling and nauseating.

Stew and I have reached what I hope is a lasting peace. In the wake of our argument about Vegas, Stewart suggested a compromise: What if he and Kiwi did the same kind of trip that Scott and I were planning? No plane travel. Just an Airbnb—within driving distance—in a place that holds no special significance. And I could go away first. This seemed reasonable to me, and I started looking forward to my weekend with Scott without letting my mind veer toward Stewart's upcoming trip with Kiwi.

It's not exactly even steven, though. Daniel and Nate are at camp during my trip, but they'll be back home when Stewart is gone. *It'll be better this way,* I think. I can avoid maternal guilt when I'm with Scott, and when Stewart is with Kiwi, the kids will distract me from my jealousy.

"Are you sure you aren't running away from home?" Stewart asks when he sees what I've packed.

"It's only two bags. And my guitar." I've asked Scott to bring his bongos, too. I have a fantasy of the two of us jamming together as we drink rosé and watch the sun set. Stewart lifts my suitcase and backpack, and I follow him with the guitar. "Do you have a date with Kiwi tonight?"

"Yeah, she's driving to Brooklyn for a change." As he opens the trunk, he sees my face and adds, "Don't worry. She's not coming over here—I got a hotel."

I feel sheepish. "You didn't have to do that," I say, not really meaning it. "It seems kind of silly with the kids and me away."

"Well, it's already booked. I doubt I could cancel now."

We listen to an early Mitch Hedberg stand-up routine as we drive. *It takes forever to cook a baked potato in the oven. Sometimes I'll just throw one in there, even if I don't want one. 'Cause by the time it's done, who knows?* It feels good to laugh together. The set ends just as we get off the Garden State Parkway. I thrum my fingers against my leg to calm my nerves. Stew notices and reaches for my restless hand.

"What are you so anxious about, baby? Do you think I'm going to punch him or something?"

"It's just weird," I say.

"Only if I do this." He pulls his hand away and starts to scratch himself, making monkey sounds. "Wooga wooga!"

I break into laughter. "You're ridiculous."

"I am," he says. "But I promise to behave."

We turn the corner onto Scott's block and I see him standing in front of his house. He assured me yesterday that Diana and the kids would be gone when I arrived, but part of me still expects him to wave us on, like a lookout warning that the Feds are inside. Instead, he ambles to the curb, his hands in his pockets with a studied nonchalance. He must be nervous, too.

Stewart gets out of the car while I'm still unbuckling my seat belt, stalling. I glance out the window and see them walking toward each other. They shake hands in the middle of the empty street.

"How ya doin', man?" I hear Scott say. I've never heard him call anyone *man* before.

"Wow, you have a deep voice," says Stew. I feel my shoulders relax and open the passenger door.

"Wouldn't it be funny if I were just putting it on?" Scott replies. He puffs up his chest in comic exaggeration.

Stew laughs affably. I can tell they're both making an extra effort to get along. I feel like the only awkward one. I stand next to Stewart, unsure of where to put my eyes.

"Let me grab your stuff," he says, saving me. He squeezes my shoulder on his way back to the car, and I look at him gratefully.

"Go ahead and put it in my trunk," says Scott, pulling out his keys. The two of them walk up the block together, Stewart holding my suitcase and guitar and Scott shouldering my backpack. I envy their shared sense of purpose and continue to stand as if my legs have been dipped in concrete. They disappear behind Scott's open trunk, and I force air in and out of my lungs. Stew comes back toward me while Scott busies himself moving fishing poles. I know he's just giving us a chance to say good-bye.

Stew hugs me tightly and kisses me on the forehead. "Have fun, baby," he says. "I love you."

A lump has formed in my throat. I *feel* loved. Stew is giving me a precious gift. And I'm giving it back to him. Freedom and security are woven together in this ordinary, audacious moment.

"I love you, too," I say. "Have fun with Kiwi. And thank you. For everything."

My husband gets into the car, leaving me with my boyfriend. Who would believe my description of this scene? Scott waves as the car passes, and Stew gives the horn a friendly tap.

———

SCOTT AND I HAVE lunch at a diner en route, and by the time we arrive in Mount Kisco, it's late afternoon. The humidity has condensed into a fine mist, not quite the consistency of drizzle. The cottage Scott booked is smaller than it looked in the pictures, and he didn't read the fine print. There is a sink but no toilet or shower. It turns out we have to run into the host's house to use the bathroom.

"I'm so sorry, Molly," he tells me, flopping down on the sagging futon that serves as both couch and bed. "This place kind of sucks."

"It's fine," I say cheerfully. My mother would be proud of my can-do spirit. "Let's turn on the air conditioner. And look at this view!" The vista is truly spectacular. An entire wall of the cottage is made of windows, facing out over an expanse of green lawn, with woods beyond and the foothills of the Catskills in the distance.

Scott turns his head to look but doesn't get up from his place on the futon. "Very pretty," he says, still sounding forlorn. "Like you."

He's giving me his bedroom eyes, but I'm not ready to jump into sex. "Why don't you grab your bongos from the car?" I say, unzipping my guitar case.

Our jam session feels lackluster, and it lasts less than ten minutes. Scott and I have sex on the futon. Afterward, I dash to the host's house to avoid a UTI. We order falafel for delivery and drink the wine I brought. We loll on pillows and binge-watch *Comedians in Cars Getting Coffee.*

I'm refilling our plastic cups when I notice my phone buzzing on the end table. It's lit up with a Seamless notification: *Your order from Kiku Sushi will arrive between 8:50 and 9:00 p.m.* I stare at the message, trying to make sense of it. It must be a mistake. The kids are at camp. Who could be ordering sushi for delivery?

And then I realize: Stewart is home. With Kiwi.

Scott sees my face. "What's wrong, Beautiful?"

"I'm sorry," I say, still looking at the phone. "I have to call Stew."

I put down the cups so forcefully that some wine sloshes onto the table. I grab my phone and walk outside, closing the door without looking at Scott. The grass is cool and prickly beneath my bare feet. Shaking from head to foot, I dial Stew's number. He picks up after a couple of rings.

"What's up, baby? Everything okay?"

"Your sushi order is on its way. I just got a notice on my phone."

He laughs as if this is a great joke. "Thanks, but you didn't have to call. I'm sure the delivery guy will ring the bell."

My subtle attempts at passive aggression aren't getting through to him. It's just as well. I feel neither subtle nor passive.

"What are you doing at the house?" I ask. And then, before waiting for an answer: "You brought her to our *home*?"

Stewart is silent for a beat. "Whoa," he finally says. He lowers his voice, and I know he's shielding her from my rage. "You *told* me I could bring her over. Remember?"

"Like FUCK I did!" I shout. I want to make sure Kiwi can hear me on the other end of the line. *Where are they right now?* I wonder. *The living room? The guest room? Our bed? No. Stewart wouldn't dare.*

My question is answered by the sound of Stewart's feet on tile, the bang of a screen door. He's left Kiwi in the kitchen and has gone to the back porch so she can't hear our argument. Instead, the neighbors will get front-row seats.

"And I quote," he says, his own voice rising now, too. *"You didn't have to get a room,* you said. *It's silly,* you said. So I called the hotel, and they let me cancel."

The self-righteous ground is crumbling beneath me and my legs go weak. I plop down cross-legged on the grass, welcoming the sharp blades that reach into my shorts and scrape my upper thighs.

"I just said that to be nice," I explain. "I didn't mean it. You should have known I don't want her at our house."

"You're right," he says sarcastically. "I'm so sorry I didn't read your mind when you said the opposite of what you meant."

"Fuck you. Just get her out of my house and book a hotel." I hang up the phone. Then I lie down and close my eyes, letting tears trickle into my ears. A wedge of light falls over me, and I turn my head to see Scott in the doorway.

"Hey there, Beautiful," he says. "What happened?"

I don't feel like talking about it, but I tell him anyway. Sort of. I omit the part where I told Stew he could cancel the hotel. I don't want Scott seeing things from his perspective.

"That's really shitty," he says. He's sitting next to me now, plucking idly at the grass. I feel a pang of shame for painting Stew in a negative light. But it feels good to have Scott firmly on my side. He adds, "Not nearly as shitty as what Diana's up to, but still. Shitty."

"What's Diana doing? Didn't she take the kids somewhere so we could go away together?"

He groans and keeps his eyes on the ground. "Yeah. But I didn't tell you where she went. I didn't want to ruin our time together with my problems." He takes a blade of grass between his thumb and middle finger and flicks it into the darkness.

A bubble of anxiety surfaces in my throat. "Tell me," I say.

He glances at me but turns away before he speaks. "She took the kids to California. To meet Rick."

I am mute, trying to process this information. There is only one way to interpret it.

"She wants to move there, to be closer to him. She asked me for a divorce a few days ago." He continues to study the grass.

"Oh God, Scott. I'm so sorry." I hope he can't see the places my mind is going. *Is this why Diana wanted to open the marriage? To find herself a new husband before leaving Scott?*

"Don't be sorry," he says. And then, as if reading my thoughts: "Our marriage has been dying for a long time."

We sit in silence for a few beats. I want to be present for Scott's sake, but my brain careens forward, exploring one dire scenario after another.

"But wait. She can't move the kids across the country, can she?"

"Diana always gets what she wants," he says. "There's not much I can do about it."

"That's insane!" I say, stunned by his attitude of defeat. "Of *course* there are things you can do. You need a good lawyer, for starters."

"You're probably right." He turns to look me full in the face. "I'm so lucky to have you in my life."

I want to say the same thing back to him, but I can't. My head is spinning, and a migraine is forming behind my eyes.

"C'mon," he says, standing up and reaching out his hand to pull me to my feet. "Let's not waste any more time talking about Stew and Diana. Fuck them."

That night, I try to go to sleep as the little spoon, nestled inside Scott's arms. Instead, I lie awake for a long time as Scott snores softly into my hair. When he rolls onto his other side, I creep out of bed and grope along the table to find my phone. It's two fifteen.

Hi, baby. I doubt you're still awake, but I need to write you anyway. I'm sorry for freaking out before. It wasn't fair of me to give you mixed messages and then expect you to know how I felt.

I hit Send. The appearance of three dots surprises me, and I grip the phone with both hands, waiting to see Stew's reply.

I'm the one who should be sorry. It was stupid of me to think that an offhanded remark was permission to have Kiwi at our house. You were right to be upset.

I reread his message a few times. *Wow,* I respond. *We're getting much better at fighting. Don't you think so?*

Haha. I agree.

I hesitate before telling him the other thing that's weighing on my mind. But I can't keep it to myself.

Diana asked Scott for a divorce.

Oh, shit. Is he okay?

It's hard to tell. I'm just so glad that you and I are solid.

Always, my baby. Always.

Good night, Stewbie. I love you.

Sleep well, Suitcase. I love you, too. Fuckloads.

I WAKE UP TO the morning light coming through the curtain-less windows. It's already hot and hazy when we head out with our fishing poles. Despite the humidity, Scott wears his typical flannel and jeans, with heavy fishing boots. When we arrive at the water's edge, which is swarming with insects, I look down at my bare legs and open-toed sandals and feel unprepared.

I shift my weight from one foot to the other and swat at mosquitoes and gnats while Scott opens his tackle box. It's hyper-organized in a way that seems discordant with the Scott I know. I watch him attach a lure to the line, his fingers nimble and sure. And then he hands the pole to me.

"Here you go, Beautiful," he says.

He coaches me on how to cast. The first time I try, I forget to push the button, or let go of the button, or whatever one is supposed to do when casting. Scott laughs. He steps onto the bank where I'm standing, moving easily over the slippery rocks, and stands behind me, showing me what to do. His small, smooth hands—feminine hands that contrast with his whiskey smell and the deep growl of his voice—cover mine. Scott guides and I follow, and the line sails far out into the dark blue water. He is adept at this, at fishing, and his competence is sexy. I focus on the feel of his hands and the smooth motion of our arms, working in concert, and try to forget that Scott's life is falling apart.

A FEW WEEKS LATER, Stewart goes on a hiking trip in the Poconos with Kiwi. I hear the garage door open at around eleven p.m. on Sunday, after the kids are asleep, and I'm glad Stew will find me here—sitting on our bed, folding laundry and watching TV. This relaxed yet productive pose is the image I want to convey, and it's almost accurate. I've had a good couple of days. On Friday, I had drinks with Jessie. On Saturday morning, I boxed. Then Susan came over and we cooked dinner for the kids, drank wine, played guitar. Today I took the boys back-to-school shopping. We ordered pizza and watched a movie. In brief snatches, I'd remember: *Stewart is with Kiwi now.* But I haven't dwelled on it. Instead, I've focused on my own life, on the moment I'm living rather than the one I'm not. I feel proud of how well I've done.

So I'm surprised to feel my throat tighten as Stewart begins to answer my simple question:

"How was it?"

"We didn't go hiking—it was too rainy," he says. "So we went outlet shopping, and I bought some shoes. And then we went bowling." He continues on, his voice animated. Their weekend was very domestic, he tells me. Kiwi had her period, and everything in the Airbnb was white, making sex more cautious than passionate. Then Stew spilled guacamole on the couch, and they had to spend forty minutes trying to get the spot out. He describes these events as negatives, but this type of at-home-and-in-it-together scenario is what I've always craved from him. I've come to think of domestic tasks as something I do separately from my husband, something that Stewart avoids at all costs. By the time Stew gets to the part about making dinner with Kiwi—and that he peeled the potatoes—I'm in tears.

He stops talking. "Why are you crying?" he asks, genuinely dumbfounded.

It's the damn potatoes.

I flash back to our session in Evelyn's office, over three years ago—*Why do you avoid being at home, Stewart?* I guess Kiwi doesn't make him feel like he's doing everything wrong. I guess when he's with her, his aversion to domesticity lifts like a sheet on a clothesline, billowing lightly in the breeze.

When I voice these guesses to Stewart, he laughs. "Oh, baby," he says. "It's not like that at all." According to Stew, their conversation around the potatoes went something like this:

You're doing it wrong, Kiwi said.

Then you do it, he countered, offering her the peeler.

I'm doing something else. Just do it right.

His reenactment of the potato-preparation scene makes me laugh. I have to admit, I admire Kiwi's no-nonsense approach to making Stewart do his share, her refusal to accept any bullshit excuses about why he can't or shouldn't or won't.

As if reading my mind, Stewart says, "To be honest, Kiwi has helped me understand a lot of things about our marriage. Like why you've been angry at me. I know I get defensive about it, but you're right that I don't help around the house enough." He reaches for my hand. "And I'm sorry for that. I'll try to do better."

I wish I could hug Kiwi. Maybe I don't need to meet her after all. We seem to have a good thing going, and she clearly has my back. Why rock the boat?

"You know," I say. "I'm learning about our marriage through

Scott, too. There are so many ways in which the two of you are different. And it makes me appreciate you more."

"I like the sound of that." Stew laughs. "How so?"

"Well, for one, Scott hates his job. It's just work for him, but I love that you're passionate about what you do. And also, it might be hard sometimes, but you and I talk things through with each other. Scott and Diana don't do that."

Stew looks down and takes my hand in his. "I might regret admitting this, but I appreciate how you *get* me to talk. Kiwi doesn't do that. Even if I know she's angry about something, she'll never tell me what it is. It can be kind of a relief, because avoiding shit is my style, too." He raises his eyes to meet mine. They're shining with moisture. I've seen Stewart cry only three times: when his father died and after the birth of each of our children. "But what you and I have is special. You're my person, baby."

"And you're mine," I whisper back.

That night, Stewart and I lie in our bed, hands still clasped, talking in the dark. For perhaps the first time ever, we talk freely and openly about love—how, despite the inevitable challenges, he loves Kiwi and I love Scott; how love morphs and evolves and differs from one situation to the next; how our love for other people only seems to make us love each other more.

"*No falling in love* is such an unrealistic rule," I say.

"Yeah, it is," Stew says, laughing. "But we didn't know that ten years ago."

"We didn't know a lot of things," I say.

"True." Neither of us speaks for a few moments, and I listen to our synchronized breathing in the silence.

"Maybe we only need one rule," I say, turning onto my side to face him. "Let's just promise to be honest with each other, and then help the other person process whatever emotions come up."

"I like that rule," he says, reaching to touch my hair.

I wriggle toward him so that our hips are touching. I snake my foot around his leg.

"I might even let you call me *cunt* during sex," I whisper.

He laughs. "Not necessary. I can get that kink elsewhere."

"Does Kiwi like it?" I ask.

"Are you sure you want to know?"

I stop and consider my answer. "I don't want a lengthy description, but yeah, I do."

"Okay," he says. "Sometimes."

"Cool," I say. And I mean it. I'm happy that Stew is getting his needs met. And that I don't have to change my boundaries for him. Is this how compersion begins?

He smiles at me in the dark and strokes my hair. Then he kisses me. Gently. Slowly. He lightly touches the skin below my belly button with his fingertips. I shiver and he stops.

"I want you to take your time coming tonight, okay?"

I nod.

"That's my good girl," he says.

CHAPTER 18

ONE MORNING IN MID-OCTOBER, I'm listening to a podcast on my way home from the gym. Nate has started seventh grade and insists on taking the subway to school by himself, so on days that I don't have workshops, I revel in my unscheduled hours. Ira Glass is interrupted by a buzz, and I see my parents' number on my phone.

"What's up?" I say, expecting my mother's voice.

I hear a low cough on the other end. "Hi, Molly. It's Dad. Is this a good time?"

Underneath his cheerful veneer, he sounds tired. I know in my bones that something is wrong. "Is everything okay?" I ask.

"Oh, yes and no," he says with a forced laugh. "Your mother is in the hospital." This nothing-to-worry-about-it's-just-life-or-death shtick is typical of my father. I want to reach through the thousand miles that separate us and shake him.

"What happened?" I hope my tone will convince him not to sugarcoat it.

"Well, she's been having some bathroom issues." I roll my eyes. My father can't handle any discussion of bodily functions. I'll need to be more specific in my line of questioning.

"Are we talking about a bladder infection? Or her urinary tract?"

"Oh no, nothing like that," he says, probably grateful that I didn't suggest a prolapsed uterus. "Just some constipation."

"Constipation doesn't land you in the hospital, Dad."

He seems relieved that I've said this. "That's what I thought. So when she was complaining of stomach pain, I didn't think much of it." Now I recognize the key emotion in his voice: guilt. "But in the middle of the night, she told me to call 911. They're doing some sort of scan now. I just came home to walk Hugo. Hopefully we'll know what it is in a few hours."

"I'm coming, Dad."

"Oh, that's not necessary," he says, then backpedals. "Although it would certainly cheer your mother up to know you're on your way."

"I'll book a flight right now."

IN THE CAB ON my way to LaGuardia, knowing that my father rarely asks the right questions and doesn't have a cell phone to keep in touch with me anyway, I call the hospital and speak with the attending physician. My mother has a twisted bowel and needs emergency surgery. My next move is to google *twisted bowel and Parkinson's* on my phone. I'm led down a rabbit hole of all the health issues that derive from advanced Parkinson's disease: digestive problems, falling, pneumonia, even hallucinations and dementia. I send Stewart links to articles about the direst possibilities, and he texts me back: *You're going to drive yourself crazy, baby. Maybe listen to some music instead?*

I know he's right. But music feels like a betrayal of my mother's suffering. On the plane, I listen to white noise on my headphones and close my eyes. My fear refuses to subside. *My mother will die,* I think. *If not now, then soon.*

It's close to five when I arrive at the hospital, the place where I was born. I find my father in the lobby, asleep with his chin against his chest, snoring lightly. A thick historical biography is in his lap, his finger inserted in the pages to mark his place. His beard is completely white now, and his thinning hair is combed over to cover the bald expanse of his scalp. My hand is poised to touch his shoulder, but I hesitate to wake him. He opens his eyes, sitting up with a start.

"You're here!" he says with a mix of shock and relief.

"Hi, Dad." I bend over awkwardly to hug him.

"Hi, kiddo," he says, patting my back. "It was good of you to come."

A FEW HOURS LATER, when my mother wakes up from her anesthesia and sees me, tears appear in her eyes, but she is unable to smile, let alone speak. It's been almost twenty-four hours since her last dose of Sinemet, the Parkinson's wonder drug. Without medication, her body keeps her prisoner. Even if we bring her pills from home, she won't be able to swallow them, and I hound the resident on duty to go through the necessary protocols to add levodopa to her IV drip. Once the magic ingredient enters her bloodstream, it will take a few more hours to set her free.

I send my father home to rest, using their old white Lab as an excuse. "You go take care of Hugo, Dad. I'll stay with Mom tonight." I look away as he kisses her on the forehead, whispers in her ear.

After finding a blanket and pillow in the closet, I settle into the reclining chair next to my mother's bed. I watch her face for signs of discomfort and hold her hand when she winces.

Throughout the night, various nurses move in and out of the room to check my mother's vital signs. Some of them turn on the lights. When they speak to her, I intervene on her behalf.

"She has Parkinson's," I explain again and again, shocked that this information isn't front and center on her chart. "She missed a bunch of doses of her medication when she was in surgery, and she can't really speak or move until it kicks in again." My mother's eyes find mine, and I see her gratitude in them.

By dawn, she manages a hoarse whisper: "Molly."

"I'm here, Mom," I say, squeezing her hand. "I'm here."

FOR THE NEXT COUPLE of days, I keep vigil from the reclining chair and pop Excedrin to stave off the migraine that's building behind my eyes. My father comes and goes but has difficulty performing the tasks I've taken on. My mother's voice is still weak, and my dad's poor hearing makes it hard for her to get his attention. I, on the other hand, am hyperattuned to her every need. I press the Call button for the nurse when she needs to pee. I readjust her pillows every hour. I swab her mouth with a sponge dipped in ice water. It's clear my mother prefers my ministrations to my father's rough attempts, and I send him home every afternoon to "take care of Hugo."

On the third day, my mom frets about missing her book club. "I'm afraid they'll worry about me."

"Should I send a group email?" I ask.

"But you don't have their addresses."

"I'll log in to your Gmail. What's your password?"

My mother is astounded that I can do this. After I send the book club message, she asks if I can see who has written to her over the past few days. I've already texted everyone in the family—my sister and aunts, nephews, and cousins—but now I scan her inbox for other names.

And then I see it: an email from Jim. A quick glance down my mother's list of messages shows that he writes her quite a bit. The subject lines say things like *Too funny!* and *Are you back yet?*

"Do you want me to read it to you?" I ask, hesitating. "He sent it yesterday."

"Sure," she says. I look at my mother's frail body, dwarfed by the hospital bed. I don't suppose their exchanges are very racy anymore—if they ever were—so I click on his message and read.

Hello, dearie! I tried calling this morning but there was no answer and the machine is full. Hope you're doing okay. Let me know if you and Phil want to get brunch next weekend!
xo J

"That's nice," my mother says. I scrutinize her smile like an art student examining the *Mona Lisa*. "Could you write him back and let him know what happened? Tell him I'll call once I'm home. I'm going to close my eyes for a few minutes now, if that's okay."

"Of course, Mom."

I follow my mother's instructions, and hit Send just as my dad walks in. I gasp as if I'm participating in a cover-up. I have to remind myself that my father knows all about Jim. They still get together for brunch, for goodness' sake.

But now I have an idea.

"Hey, Dad," I whisper, nodding toward my sleeping mother. "I think I'll go back to the house and take a shower."

"Good idea." He hands me the keys to his Honda. "You don't need to put the key in the ignition. Just keep it in your pocket." I've been driving his "new" car on every visit home for the past three years, and my own car operates the same way.

"Yes, Dad. I know."

I FIND MYSELF ALONE at my parents' house, the house I grew up in. When I let Hugo out of the back room, he wags his tail in ecstasy at the presence of another living being.

"I get it, Hugo," I say, petting his white fur. "This house feels strange when it's empty." He follows me up the stairs and plops down on the cushion my parents keep for him in their bedroom.

My eyes fall on my mother's desk. It's the same shape and color as a kidney bean—three curved drawers of increasing depth on each side, plus a narrow one in the middle—so my mother calls it her kidney-shaped desk. When my sister or I needed a pen to do homework, or when my father was searching for the checkbook or a stamp, she would shout up the stairs, *Look in the kidney-shaped desk!*

I think back to our last night at the retreat in North Carolina. After we talked—with minimal detail—about our respective threesomes, my mom told me a few other tidbits. How she also used to cry after an orgasm. How on the night my dad's father died, she was on a date with Jim and still felt guilty about it. But I want to know things she won't say. I want to know things she can't admit, even to herself.

I start with the shallowest drawer on the left. Aside from dust and a few paper clips, I find a little blue book. Inside the front cover, I'm surprised to see my own handwriting—a careful cursive, the letters rounded with circles over the *i*'s, marking it as an archive of my middle school years:

> *Happy Birthday, Mom!*
> *You are the best mommy in the world and I love you more than anything.*
> *Love, Molly*

Subsequent pages are in my mother's hand. In them, she writes about her upcoming sabbatical from teaching:

> *I want to take art and/or music classes and/or Tai-chi lessons—something to take me out of my head and away from the "shoulds" that have so shaped my life.*

I know all about these *shoulds*: obligations derived from marriage and motherhood and existing in the world as a woman. But the uncertainty of the *and/or*s fills me with a sadness that's difficult to name. To search without knowing what you're looking for. *This?* my mother seems to ask. *Will this and/or this make me whole?* I close the book.

I move down to one of the deeper drawers and gently lift a stack of papers. There are photographs, birthday cards, and aerograms, delicate as an onion's outer skin. When I see Jim's name on a return address, my heart quickens. I pause and pull out my phone.

"Hey, baby," I say when Stewart picks up. "I'm snooping at my parents' house, and I'm about to read my mom's letters. Do you think I'm a horrible person?"

There's no turning back, and we both know it. But he understands that I'm looking for permission.

"Go for it," he tells me. "And don't worry. I'm sure Daniel and Nate look through our shit, too."

"Thanks," I say. "I'm holding a letter from Jesus Christ right now. I'll let you know if I find anything good."

He laughs. "I'm counting on it."

Crouched on the floor in my parents' bedroom, I read through all the letters from Jim I can find. I'm disappointed. I thought they'd be sexier. Instead, they're all about acting gigs and Mahikari teachings.

In one letter, Jim refers to a trip my mother told me about as we drove to the Charlotte airport after our retreat. She and Jim had traveled together from Chicago to California to take their second Mahikari initiation, a deepening of their commitment to the practice. My mother remembers the trip as romantic, but she also told me it was chaste. By that point, she was seeing Buddha, who had forbidden her relationship with Jim. As a sensei, my mom explained, Buddha was used to giving orders. My mother, ever obedient, complied.

In another letter, Jim responds to my mom's misgivings about Mahikari, early doubts I'd been unaware of. As far as I knew, she was a devoted member from 1978 until the day in 1994 when she typed Mahikari into the brand-new World Wide Web and saw articles with titles like "How to Escape a Cult" and "Mahikari of America Sued for Fraud." But Jim's letter had been written at least ten years before that.

I discussed your questions with a doshi at the Center, he writes. *He suggests that you think of your struggles with Mahikari as similar to walking a tightrope.*

If the objective is to provide comfort, this seems like a strange metaphor. I picture my mother, as deathly afraid of heights as I am, high above solid ground in the immaterial world of Mahikari, afraid of what might happen if she steps off the dangerously thin wire that holds her aloft.

Still, in his letters, Jim calls my mother "Dearie," just as he did in his email. There is affection here, and friendship, and respect.

I move on through the pile to look for letters from Buddha, carefully sifting through the airmail envelopes until I see two or three with his surname. The contents are even more boring. Buddha has the flu. He's looking for a new job. His children are well. Granted, English isn't his first language, so his letters are understandably limited. I keep hunting—for what exactly, I'm not sure—and land upon a pile of photos.

There are two snapshots of my mom and Buddha in an airport, taken separately, as if they had each turned the camera on the other. I recognize Buddha's shaggy hair and square jaw. Although I never thought about it as a kid, I see now that he's a handsome man.

But I can't take my eyes off the picture of my mother. She is radiant in a bright blue blouse, a flowered skirt, and white sandals that match her purse. Her slim, pretty legs are crossed at the ankles, and she leans her cheek against one hand, her lively eyes looking at the man taking the picture. Her smile shows even, white teeth. I try to guess her age in the photo. It must have been taken on another trip I vaguely remember, the year I was fourteen and she was forty-four, the age I am now. She went to Japan to take her third and final Mahikari initiation—and to see Buddha, she told me as we drove through the North Carolina mountains. Toward the end of the trip, Buddha booked a fancy Tokyo hotel for the two of them. But by then, my mother had met Buddha's wife—he'd been cheating all along—and she was done. Besides, Buddha went in a different spiritual direction after his return to Japan. He disavowed Mahikari and became a Jehovah's Witness.

BACK AT THE HOSPITAL, I don't mention my search through the kidney-shaped desk. Instead, I update my parents on phone calls they missed and how many times Hugo pooped. Later, my father mutes the Northwestern-Nebraska football game, and the three of us play a cooperative version of Super Boggle, my father creating long lists of words dictated by my mother and me so my mom doesn't have to write. Gone are the days of my father's famed victory laps after winning a dog-eat-dog game of Hearts or Scrabble. The two of them play Super Boggle almost every night, and sheets of paper—the relics of their past games, including a triumphant four-hundred-pointer—fill the box.

After our game, my father goes home, taking this last chance to get a solid night's sleep before I fly back to New York in the morning. I walk with him to his car, and in the solitude of the hospital's parking garage, he tells me, "This past week is the first time I've looked at your mother and seen an old woman."

I think of another photo I saw earlier that day, as I left behind the kidney-shaped desk and idly flipped through my parents' wedding album. It struck me because it was the only image that didn't look posed. In it, my mother and father sit outside on a blanket. My mother's back, elegant in her gown, is to the camera. My father leans on an elbow and looks at her, captivated.

According to my mom, my dad appreciated both Jim's and Buddha's presence in her life. They filled a need my father didn't— the pursuit of a spiritual path, I suppose. But my dad never seemed to feel threatened, and clearly there was no reason to. He is, after all, the one who plays Super Boggle with my mother every evening and rushes to her side in the night.

I return to the hospital room and look at my phone while my mother rests.

"Are you reading love letters?" she asks, her eyes still closed. I think about my snooping and feel a jolt of guilt.

I'm reading texts from Stew (*Our bed feels empty without you*), from Scott (*How's your mother?*), from Nate (*Will you be home tomorrow, Mom?*), and more from Nina, Jessie, Susan, and other friends who know that my mother is in the hospital and are checking on me.

"I guess I am," I answer. If these aren't love letters, what are?

She opens her eyes and turns to face me. "Did I tell you about the email Buddha sent me? It was a few months ago."

"No," I say. "You didn't. What did he write?"

"You can find it, can't you? In my account?"

I log in to my mother's Gmail and type his name in the search bar, then open the single message that appears. It's only a couple of lines, but it's so moving that I have to catch my breath. I look over at my mom. Her eyes are closed again, and she has that same *Mona Lisa* smile on her face.

"Can you read it aloud to me?" she says. "I want to hear it again."

"*Mary,*" I read. "*You were in my dream last night. And you were beautiful.*"

CHAPTER 19

OVER THE NEXT FEW months, my mother is in and out of the hospital. During her recovery from the twisted bowel, she falls and breaks her clavicle. Persistent "bathroom issues," as my father continues to call them, put pressure on her digestive tract—and she ends up with appendicitis.

I travel between LaGuardia and O'Hare several times. I give my father respite from the constant care she requires and arrange for help when I'm gone. I meet with my mother's various doctors, trying to solve the problem of her failing body.

I want to fix things. If only I can procure the right combination of goods and services, I believe, enlisting the help of Amazon Prime and visiting nurses, I can save my mother from the perils of old age. I can save her from the certainty of death.

It's not until the first week of January that I schedule a session with Mitchell. With all of the back-and-forth, perhaps I really haven't had time. Or perhaps I don't have the energy to look inward. A dull ache in my head has been my constant companion for months. It looms like a shadow.

When I sit down on Mitchell's couch, exhaling heavily, he asks right away: "How is your head?"

A laugh escapes my lips, and I can taste its bitterness. "I guess it's obvious," I say.

Mitchell nods. "Maybe we can use your migraine to guide

today's session. Do you recall when you first started feeling it? Or any patterns when it gets particularly bad?"

"I remember that I got one the first time my mom was in the hospital." Mitchell knows this much about my life in recent months. My mother's health has been my excuse for every cancellation. "And I get a migraine every time I'm back home. But I think I'm just exhausted."

He jots down a note without speaking.

"Also, Scott is going through a stressful time. He and his wife told their kids about the divorce on Christmas Eve."

Mitchell points his pen right at my heart. "And how does Scott's stress impact *you*?"

"He's been calling me a lot," I say. "Usually when he's doing laundry." I'm not sure why I include this detail, but it seems important to me. *Hi, Beautiful,* he always says. I can hear the whirring of the machine, the echoey stillness of the basement, the profound sadness in his voice.

Mitchell just looks at me, a tacit reminder that I haven't answered his question.

"I feel bad for him. Diana is being so impulsive. I mean, she's planning on marrying this guy she met only a year ago. She has this vision of moving to Malibu with the kids, but now their daughter wants to stay with Scott and finish high school in New Jersey. And their son is taking it hard. He's only nine." I pause, and Mitchell remains silent, making me self-conscious about what I'm not saying. "I know all his family drama affects me, but I'm not sure how to explain it."

"Take your time," he says. "Let your feelings come to the surface. Maybe closing your eyes would help."

I shut my eyes and take a deep breath. Several images jockey for position in my mind. I see Scott's son—from a picture on Diana's

Facebook page—dressed for a Little League game. And then I see Nate, standing in the hallway in his pajamas, still wanting me to sing him a song and tuck him in at bedtime. I see Scott's sad eyes. I remember another of his phone calls, late at night—from a bar this time, not the laundry room—and Scott's drunken voice asking me, *Will you ever leave him, Molly? He'll never love you like I do.* He texted the next morning to apologize, blaming the booze, and I set it aside. But now my head burns. I keep my eyes closed, and words pour out like water to quell the flames.

"Scott wants me to meet his son. But I can't. It sounds crazy, but it makes me feel like I'm cheating on Nate. And I'm afraid what Scott really wants is for me to leave Stewart and marry him, to be a mother to his children. And I can't. I have my own family. I love Stewart. I love the life we have together. But I love Scott, too. I really do. I just don't know if he's going to accept reality."

When I finish my monologue, I open my eyes and look at Mitchell.

"I see where the headaches are coming from," he says. "Straight-A Molly strikes again."

I start to protest, but he's right. I'm trying to please, to take care of, to save—my parents as well as Scott. How could I not have seen it before? I'm not sure whether to laugh or to scream. I sit with my mouth agape, unable to decide what to do with it.

Mitchell reads my face. "Let's try something," he says.

He pulls out the chair across from his desk and positions it in front of me. Then he takes a pillow from the couch and puts it on the chair. He reaches for my hat from the coatrack and places it on top of the pillow.

"This is Straight-A Molly."

I laugh. "Okaaay."

"You're Real Molly. True Molly. I want you to talk to Straight-A

Molly. Your perfect self that has been doing everything she can to take care of everyone else since she was a little girl. She needs to hear from you right now. What do you want to say to her?"

I look at the pillow with the hat, and I can see her. Straight-A Molly is talking on the phone with Scott, helping him through his divorce. She is flying to Chicago every other weekend to take care of her mother. She's kissing Martina's breasts. She's juggling two children and a job while gulping down her poisonous anger. She is joining Mahikari to make her mother happy. And there she is, Straight-A Molly at age eight, her pink-framed glasses poking out from under a mop of sandy hair as she bends over her workbook with a sharpened pencil, determined to do it all.

I want to pick her up and hold her, and so I do. Her hat falls off, but it doesn't matter. I cradle her in my arms, rocking her back and forth. I tell my "perfect" self that she doesn't have to please others to have her needs met, that *I'll* take care of her. I'm not sure who's crying now—True Molly or Straight-A Molly. We're wet with the same tears.

"How's your head now?" Mitchell asks gently when my weeping subsides.

"Better," I say, still clutching the pillow as I reach for a tissue. "But I feel so frustrated. One day, I'm sure I'm making progress. And then I realize I'm learning the same goddamn lesson all over again."

As I blow my nose, Mitchell looks to the ceiling, either giving me privacy to wipe away my snot or allowing some wisdom to formulate. I'm grateful for the former but hoping for the latter.

"Don't be fooled, Molly," he says finally. "It's like being on a spiral staircase—the view feels the same, but in truth, you're a bit higher up."

———

AS I LIE AWAKE in bed that night, I'm visited by a childhood memory.

I was six years old. I'd slept over at my friend Gretchen's house, and during the night, a blizzard hit. The snow was so deep that the plows couldn't get through, and I stayed over for a second night. But by the third day, I wanted to go home. Gretchen's mom wasn't exactly mean, but her stern, accented voice scared me, and Gretchen had to practice violin for several hours every day, whether I was there or not. They didn't have orange juice at their house—only grape juice, which gave me diarrhea. And we ate the same spaghetti for dinner two nights in a row. It tasted funny, not at all like my mom's spaghetti.

I called my parents and cried on the phone.

Daniel and Nate never had sleepovers that young. It makes me doubt my memory, but my recollection jibes with the timing of the biggest blizzard in Chicago history. The one I remember must have been in January 1979—thirty-nine years ago. And still, even at an age that now strikes me as too young to be away from home, I never dreamed that anyone would come to my rescue. I would need to figure it out on my own. To take care of myself.

Gretchen lived just a few blocks away, but snow was piled so high that only the tops of cars peeked above the glittering expanse of white. Porch steps were hidden, and the top of each house seemed too low for regular-size people to live in. But when my father heard me crying on the phone, he said, "Hang on. I'll be there soon."

I put on my boots and coat, my mittens and hat, and sat roasting in that getup as I waited. Gretchen was practicing violin upstairs, and as I looked out the living room window, I felt an anticipation like Christmas Eve.

And then I saw my dad.

His beard was laced with snow, and he trudged down the center of the buried street, carving a passageway with gloved hands, a floating torso. Next I remember sitting atop my father's heroic shoulders as he walked toward home in the path created by his forward trek. The sound of his labored breath, the puffs of visible air floating before his face, the feel of his hands securing my dangled legs as he bent forward into the blowing drifts, taking me home, keeping me safe.

In the drowsy haze that separates memory from dream, my father lifts my little-girl self from his shoulders and hands her to grown-up me. I'm big enough to carry her now, to mother her, to take care of her needs. I hold my sweet little Straight-A Molly close as I fall asleep.

CHAPTER 20

SCOTT'S DIVORCE GOES THROUGH at breakneck speed. He decides not to seek legal counsel and contests nothing. Diana will be moving his son to California.

On the other end of his phone calls, I hold my tongue. His passivity baffles me, but I restrain myself from offering to hire a lawyer on his behalf. The lyrics of a new song come to me in their entirety, and I write them down, put them to chords with a strumming pattern I borrow from the Mountain Goats, one of Scott's favorite bands:

> *In the end we both know the point can't possibly be*
> *That I can't save you, and you can't save me*

DIANA'S ATTORNEY DRAWS UP the divorce agreement, and Scott signs it just before Valentine's Day. *Let me take you out,* I text. We haven't seen each other in a few weeks. I've encouraged him to take this time, to give his attention to his kids. Plus, he's looking for his own apartment. I know he's worried about affording the rent, so I book our hotel room and make the dinner reservations. On the subway, on my way to meet Scott in midtown, I pull out the Valentine's Day card I bought at the pharmacy and stare at the blank page inside. What can I say that is entirely true? I pop in my earbuds and put Scott's most recent playlist—"Mix for Molly #5"—on shuffle. Scott enters my thoughts through my ears, as he's always done. And each song seems to give me one more piece of the truth of us.

I get to the hotel first and check in. When Scott texts from Port Authority, I go outside to wait for him, the cold air whipping my face. Soon he is walking toward me from the end of the block, his jacket too light for the weather, no hat or gloves, his hands stuffed deep into the pockets of his jeans. He keeps his head down—to shield his face from the wind, I assume. But when his eyes dart to meet mine, he smiles weakly before lowering his gaze. I feel a dull sense of foreboding in my gut as I reach out to hug him.

"Hey," he says, still not looking me in the eye. "I really need to talk to you."

"We have the whole night," I say. "Let's go up to the room."

"Do you mind if we talk out here?"

"You're acting weird," I tell him. "What's going on?"

He pulls me by the sleeve to a spot against the brick-faced wall, sheltered from the wind.

"So I moved into my own place on Saturday."

"You did? I thought you were still looking," I say, confused. "But that's great! I can't wait to see it."

He takes a deep breath, then spits out the rest quickly: "I don't want to be alone, Molly. I want to be with you but only if you can really be with me." He shakes his head. "I can't believe I'm doing this."

"Doing what?" I ask, but I know. He remains silent, his eyes down. "Are you breaking up with me?" It's unexpected and inevitable all at once. Like the way Scott kisses me.

"I don't want to, Molly. I love you. I want to be with you. But I have to know: Will you ever leave Stewart?"

I concentrate on keeping my breaths even. *In two three, out two three.* "I'm never leaving Stewart. You've known that from the beginning."

"Never, Beautiful?" His voice is rough with effort. "Not even when your kids leave?"

"Scott, I love you. *And* I love Stewart. Just because Diana messed it up doesn't mean I'm leaving my husband. Why can't we stay the way we are?"

"Because I met someone else," he mumbles.

I feel a wave rising. Before it crashes over me, I ask a measured question: "Why can't you see us both?"

The answer is in his eyes, and I know what I've been ignoring for months. Maybe since the beginning. Scott wants monogamy.

"I don't think that will work," he whispers.

I feel dizzy. I close my eyes to steady myself. When I open them again, the streetlights are too bright. I nod, but I can't speak. Instead, I turn and walk toward the hotel entrance. I need to be alone.

"Molly," Scott calls after me. "Molly, I'm sorry."

I take the elevator up to the room I'd left just fifteen minutes before. It feels small. Empty. My Valentine's Day card is peeking from the top of my bag. I pull it out and open the envelope.

I love you, Scott, I'd written. *I will always love you.*

I try to rip it up, but the cardstock paper is too thick. And anyway, ripping it won't make the words less true.

I throw myself facedown on the bed, waiting for the sobs to come. But instead, something else rises to the surface. It's my mother's voice: *Oh, sweetheart. There will be more.*

My chest is pulled into a familiar ache. It feels both good and bad. It's like the pain felt the day after a hard workout, a physical reminder that something has changed in the muscle of the heart, a sweet burn that lingers.

There will be more.

I thought my mother had meant there would be more men. More boyfriends. More exciting trysts to help me escape the realities of marriage and motherhood.

But what she really meant is this: *There will be more love.*

I remember how, on the night before Nate was born, I crept into the room where Daniel slept. My pregnant belly brushed the bars of the crib he would soon need to vacate, to make space for his little brother. I felt so sorry that my heart would need to make space as well. How could I love another child when my love for Daniel filled me to bursting?

But then a miracle happened. Nate arrived. And I loved them both.

Because love is vast. Abundant. Infinite, in fact. And the secret is this: love begets love. The more you love, the more love you have to give.

I lie on the bed in the empty hotel room and feel love coursing through me. It's painful and it's beautiful, and the pain and the beauty are part of the same thing. Yes, I love Scott. And yes, I love Stewart. And yes, there will be more. My heart is open enough to hold it all.

I put my coat on and leave the room. I take the elevator down to the lobby and step back into the cold night. Scott is gone, as I knew he would be. Perhaps I'd see him again. Perhaps not. But either way, I'd continue to love him.

I pull out my phone and call Stewart.

"Hi, baby. What's up?"

"Scott and I just broke up," I say. My voice cracks as I say this. But it's okay. I'm okay.

"Oh, baby," he says. "I'm so sorry. I was just about to leave to meet Kiwi, but I can cancel. Do you want me to?"

Stew has offered to cancel his plans with Kiwi before—on other nights when I burned with rage or cried myself to sleep. I've always steeled myself and told him to go, lied and said I'd be fine. But tonight is different. Tonight I'll love myself enough to accept Stewart's love.

"Yes," I say. "Thank you."

"Hang on," my husband tells me. "I'll be right there."

Acknowledgments

I first got the idea to write this memoir in April 2019. Since that time, I have received so much support and guidance that it's difficult to parse.

To the teachers who got me started—Michele Filgate and Heather Aimee O'Neill of Sackett Street Writers' Workshop, Emily Stone, and the folks at StoryStudio Chicago—thank you for helping me to find my writing voice and to overcome a case of impostor syndrome. I am also indebted to my fellow writers in the many workshops I attended. Your feedback and enthusiasm for my project were invaluable. Special thanks to Christie Tate for putting aside her own work to read my proposal and write my very first blurb.

To Sam Hiyate—my agent at the Rights Factory who said to me more than once, "I love it. But you have to start over"—thank you for believing in my book from the very beginning and for helping to give it shape.

To my editor, Kris Puopolo, and the team at Doubleday—thank you not only for your editorial talents and warmth but also for your willingness to take a chance on a debut author without a TikTok account. I have felt myself to be in very good hands.

To Jen Ziegler, Jake Kolton, and the Café Martin community in Park Slope—thank you for the inspiring conversations, the encouragement, and the caffeine. This book would not exist without you.

To Carey—thank you for being my one and only soul sister.

To my friends—especially Jennifer Saba, Emily Isaac, Julie Meyer, Rebecca Morrissey, Karima Hassan Hopkins, Rachel Mazor, and Maaza Mengiste—thanks to those of you who read early drafts, and to all of you for cheering me on.

To the men I've dated along the way—to those I've loved and lost, and to those who continue to love me back—I thank you all for showing me pieces of myself that might otherwise have stayed hidden.

To Michael Cohen—thank you for seeing me, for sharing your wisdom, and for helping me to patch that darn hole in my bucket.

To my parents—thank you for encouraging me to tell my story, as well as graciously allowing me to share my version of yours. Your trust and love mean the world to me.

To my children—who have taught me more about love than anyone—thank you for being the extraordinary young men that you are. I would not be myself without you. And I'm so very proud to be your mother.

To Stewart, who did not flinch when I first spoke of my idea to write this book, and who has stood by me every step of the way—thank you for being my person. I love loving you.

More: A Memoir of Open Marriage

READING GUIDE

PRE-READING

- Consider the epigraph, the quote by Audre Lorde: "The erotic is the nurturer . . . of all our deepest knowledge." What kind of self-knowledge can arise from erotic experiences?
- In the Author's Note, Molly says she consulted her journals as preparation for writing this memoir and was "shocked to discover how often I had lied to myself." Think about areas of life in which you specifically—or people in general—sometimes have a hard time admitting the truth to yourself.

PROLOGUE

- In the Prologue, Molly is confronted by her thirteen-year-old son about her open marriage. What is the most awkward conversation you've ever had (or avoided having) with your own parents or children? What is your personal philosophy regarding boundaries vs. honesty when talking with one's parents or children?

PART ONE

- In chapter 3, Molly tells her friend Jessie about her time with Matt at the karaoke party. Jessie says it sounds like Molly is "entering dangerous territory." Do you agree with Jessie? What is dangerous about this situation? Do you agree with Molly that "once in a while, it's important to do the dangerous thing"?
- In chapter 4, Stewart sleeps with his ex-girlfriend Lena. When Molly gets upset, he asks her if she wants to stop—that is, if she wants to close the marriage. She says "I don't know," but she has a hard time articulating her thoughts. What do *you* think are her reasons for wanting to keep the marriage open?
- In chapter 5, Molly accidentally sends a text meant for Stewart to Matt. Have you ever sent a text to the wrong person? What happened?

- In chapter 6, Mitchell gives Molly the "homework" of making a list of the freedoms she desires: Freedom From, Freedom to Be, Freedom to Do. Think about freedom in your own life. If you were to create a similar list, what would be on it?

PART TWO
- In chapters 7 and 8, Molly is engaged in sexual exploration with men she has met on Ashley Madison. Chapter 8 ends with these lines: "How have I arrived at this point? I'm honestly not sure. Shame will do that, smear the details until they become tolerable." What do you think is the root source of Molly's shame?
- In chapter 9, Molly goes to therapy and Mitchell tells her, "I think there's a hole in your bucket." Can you relate to this image? Discuss.
- In chapters 10 and 11, Molly starts to date Karl. What do you think appeals to her most about this relationship? Do you agree with the couple's therapist, who tells Molly and Stewart that "there are risks" to their outside relationships?
- Discuss the events of chapter 12—namely, Molly's decision to have a threesome with Karl and Martina. Did you predict how things would go after this point? Also discuss Molly's mother's advice at the end of chapter 13: "Don't waste this opportunity."

PART THREE
- In chapter 14, Molly talks about the specialness of Stewart's anniversary and birthday cards. What rituals do you maintain—or would you like to initiate—in your own relationships?
- Throughout the rest of part three, both Molly's relationship with Scott and Stewart's relationship with Kiwi become more serious. Ultimately, do you think Molly and Stewart's marriage is enhanced or threatened by these outside relationships? Discuss.
- What does the title *More* mean to you? Did you interpret the title differently after reading the last two pages?